Spiritual
Guided Imagery
for Yoga Classes

Deep Relaxation
Progressive Muscle Relaxation
Autosuggestion & Autogenic Training

Copyright © 2025 by Alida Kossack, Author
1st edition

All rights reserved.

softcover: ISBN 9781068853654
eBook: ISBN 9781068853678
alidakossack@yahoo.com
www.pranacentre.ca

German Version: 1st edition, 2025
Spirituelle Fantasiereisen für die Yogastunde
Tiefenentspannung, Progressive Muskelrelaxation,
Autosuggestion & Autogenes Training
softcover: ISBN 9781068853647
eBook: ISBN 9781068853661

book editing: Peter Michael Wiebe
English book translation: Sylvain Vallee, Regina Picco, Alida Kossack
photo of Alida Kossack: Clarisse Falcão (@sejacrisalidas)

© book cover: Alida Kossack
created by using stock graphics with Canva (www.canva.com)
creator of the graphics: anlomaja, sparklestroke, Placidplace, Mete-X

The work, including all parts, is protected by copyright. Any use without the written permission from the author is prohibited. The author is responsible for the content.

The book has been deposited with the Library and Archives Canada (LAC).
www.library-archives.canada.ca

Distribution: Amazon KDP Print und IngramSpark/Lightning Source International (LSI)

Important advice: The contents of this book have been carefully reviewed by the author based on her experience and expertise. They have proven themselves in practice. The author assumes no liability for the results. The reader should use the advice and guidance at their discretion. If you are ill or pregnant, you should always consult your doctor or therapist.

Table of Contents

Prologue	8
Chapter 1 Relaxation in Yoga Practice	10
Relaxation has to be Learned	10
Transmitter and Receiver	12
Framework Conditions	13
Competence and Experience of the Instructor	13
Trustworthiness of the Instructor	13
Room Atmosphere	14
Room Equipment	14
Preparation for the Relaxation Unit	14
Content and Process of the Relaxation Unit	16
Quality of the Relaxation Unit	18
Chapter 2 Objective of Relaxation	23
Relaxation in Today's World	24
Relaxation Techniques	25
Progressive Muscle Relaxation	25
Autogenic Training	25
Autosuggestion	27
Guided Imagery Journeys	27

Table of Contents

	Deep Relaxation	28
	Yoga	29
	QiGong	29
	TaiChi	30
Relaxation in the Yoga Class		31
	Initial Relaxation	31
	Intermediary Relaxation	33
	Final Relaxation (Deep Relaxation)	35
Effects on Body, Mind and Energy System		36
Effects on Brain Waves		38
	Gamma Waves (30–100 Hz)	39
	Beta Waves (14–30 Hz)	40
	Alpha Waves (8–14 Hz)	41
	Theta Waves (4–8 Hz)	44
	Delta Waves (0,1–4 Hz)	46

Chapter 3
Practical Part: Relaxation — 48

Relaxation Exercises in Yoga Practice	49
Directions for Reading Relaxation Instructions	50
Read-Aloud Texts for Initial Relaxation	51

Table of Contents

1. Corpse Pose	52
2. Short Progressive Muscle Relaxation	53
3. Quick Relaxation	54
3. Alternative: Body Scan	56
4. Return to the Moment	57
Read-Aloud Texts for Final Relaxation (Deep Relaxation)	58
1. Corpse Pose	59
2. Long Progressive Muscle Relaxation	60
3. Autosuggestion "Let Go and Fly"	62

Chapter 4
Practical Part: Guided Imagery Journeys	63
Guided Imagery Journeys within Yoga Classes	64
Forms of Guided Imagery Journeys	65
Closed Guided Imagery Journeys	66
Semi-Open Guided Imagery Journeys	67
Open Guided Imagery Journeys	67
Process Of Guided Imagery Journeys	68
Opening	69
Journey	69
Return	70

Table of Contents

Directions for Reading Guided Imagery Journeys	73
Read-Aloud Texts of Guided Imagery Journeys	74
Body of Light	75
Journey on a Cloud	77
Sand Bath	79
Summer Night	80
Chakra Journey	82
Full Moon	84
Yoga Nidra	86
Sacred Temple	88
Enchanted Forest	89
Bird's-eye View	91
Glowing Heart	93
Canoe Trip	95
South Sea Beach	97
Forest Walk	98
Summer Meadow	100
Waterfall	102
Winter Landscape	104
Acknowledgement of the Author	106
Books by Alida Kossack	108

THE WORLD OF REALITY HAS ITS LIMITS,
THE WORLD OF IMAGINATION IS BOUNDLESS.
(JEAN-JACQUES ROUSSEAU)

Prologue

Why are calm and relaxation so important in a yoga class? These restful moments allow us to turn away from the hustle and bustle of everyday life. They are oases of inner contemplation in which body and mind can find peace. Muscular and mental tension can now be released. We allow ourselves to temporarily disengage from the negative cycle of expectations, demands, and pressures – as a result, we reclaim our inner sanctuary.

If our body is constantly running at full speed, we lose ourselves in the stress spiral. We increasingly lose the balance between tension and relaxation that is so important for our inner equilibrium. Relaxation techniques help us to feel ourselves again and to become more aware of our real needs. They give us the necessary phases of rest and regeneration to regain our inner stability and strength.

In yoga philosophy, relaxation plays an even more significant role. **Niṣpanda** means relaxation in Sanskrit, derived from the words 'spanda' (tension) and 'ni' (without). Body and mind are free of tension. This is the basis for a contemplative mindset, which allows us access to our true self on the eight-limbed path of Ashtanga yoga:

- In the state of **Pratyahara** we calm the everyday waves of thoughts and direct our attention to inspiring and uplifting impulses.

- In the state of **Dharana**, we can bundle and focus the power of our thoughts like a laser beam. Allowing access to our higher mental power opens the gates to the hidden realms of perception, as well as to deep knowledge and wisdom.

- The state of **Dhyana**, the actual meditation, frees us from attachments to everyday wishes, desires or sensory impressions.

They dissolve like mist in the illuminating power of the morning sun. The same applies to the boundaries between body and mind, space and time. We experience a higher reality, full of calm, harmony, and peace.

- In the final stage, **Samadhi**, the last ties to the physical world are released. We are free from the limitations of separation, be it from life or from the divine life force. Instead of fear, worry and sorrow, we experience freedom, lightness, and joy of life as a constant state of mind. In oneness with the universal world soul, we experience our true nature of **Sat Chit Ananda** - perfect consciousness, infinite wisdom and unconditional bliss.

Chapter 1
Relaxation in Yoga Practice

Relaxation exercises are an essential part of a modern Hatha yoga classes. Today, yoga classes are geared to the demands of an active and performance-oriented lifestyle. Relaxation exercises allow your participants to let go both physically and mentally, and to arrive internally in the yoga class and attune themselves. It will become increasingly easier for them to detach from daily challenges, tune into and engage in their inner journey.

RELAXATION HAS TO BE LEARNED

This applies equally to you as a course leader and to your participants. As a course leader, you have a special responsibility. You are both a role model and a teacher. Before each yoga class, check whether you feel relaxed and loosened up. This will make you appear more authentic and will enable you to reach participants better.

Your participants should also be receptive to your messages to be able to get involved in the relaxation exercise. This may sound simple at first, but in practice you will face numerous questions and hurdles. However, by having a thorough understanding of the methods and how they work, you can choose the most suitable ones for your situation and achieve optimal results.

> Learning relaxation techniques requires knowledge of their content, process, and effect as well as the willingness to engage with them.

If you find relaxation easy, you will be able to teach it more easily. Through your learning process, you will also develop more patience and understanding for the learning process of your participants.

Remember that learning to open up, switch off or let go can be a long-term process and is often associated with fears and blockages. That is why not only a professional atmosphere but also trust in the course leader is important.

TRANSMITTER AND RECEIVER

Think of the example of a radio station. Likewise, during your yoga class, you offer your listeners inspiring information and messages. Here, too, you might be working with music, sounds, but above all, with your spoken words.

> These should be transmitted as clearly as possible, conveyed with as little interference as possible, but also received unfiltered.

The following framework conditions can help you optimize the quality of broadcasting and transmission. However, you have no influence on how filtered the transmitted information is received and processed in their internal system.

Yoga practice: In the relaxation sequences of your yoga class, your participants are in a more passive role of listening. They listen to your words to feel, sense or visualize them. You send them impulses and your participants decide whether it is suitable for them and which information is useful to them. You have to be on the same wavelength, so to speak. However, it is essential that your impulses are not only perceived, but also integrated into their internal system. In this way, you encourage them to develop alternative patterns of thinking and behaviour. The intention is of crucial importance here. Trust in your abilities and act with the best intentions. Then your positive and constructive impulses will be gratefully accepted.

> Be always aware that you bear a great responsibility when working with the consciousness and especially the subconscious of your participants.

FRAMEWORK CONDITIONS

Each participant strives to feel comfortable and safe. This is the only way they can open up internally and let go. In order to create the best possible framework conditions for this, the following factors should be considered.

☑ Competence and Experience of the Instructor
It is advisable to take a workshop or training in the field of relaxation techniques. This means you will not only learn a broad range of methods, but also how you can apply them in practice. The basic principles should really be understood, rehearsed and, above all, practised regularly. Even the style of speaking plays an important role. If you are a beginner, make sure to receive the most honest and constructive feedback possible from a wide target group. You will appear more confident and avoid passing on your initial insecurity to the participants. As your participants open up internally, they become more sensitive to the subtle nuances of the mood in the entire room.

☑ Trustworthiness of the Instructor
Honesty, empathy and authenticity will help your participants to trust you. Especially if you have just started working as a course leader. Know that you will always be a learner. This means that an authentic yoga teacher is also a yoga student. Are you willing to continually improve your skills and knowledge to develop further on your spiritual path? Then this effort, coupled with understanding, dedication and openness, will always connect you with your participants. It is not the illusion of a perfect yoga teacher that gives you respect and recognition, but rather the willingness to learn from those around you.

☑ Room Atmosphere

Make sure the atmosphere is pleasant and calm. You may also want to turn off the doorbell. Avoid room scents, essential oils or incense sticks, as they not only disrupt concentration but can also be disturbing. Some people may have an allergic reaction or asthmatics can have difficulty breathing. The room should invite you to switch off, let go and relax. Therefore, it should be well ventilated, tidy and open. Nobody wants to feel restricted by tripping hazards, unnecessary furniture or overloaded decorations. Also make sure to clean the floor regularly. Dust bunnies, which are caused by hair and dust, can give participants an unpleasant feeling when laying on the floor.

☑ Room Equipment

If the class is primarily focused on relaxation then the spots for your participants should be prepared in advance. This gives the room a comfortable and inviting atmosphere. Also make sure there is sufficient distance between the mats. This will prevent your hands from coming into contact with your neighbours. Equip each spot as follows:

- 1 yoga mat with a thickness of at least 4 mm
- 1 folded blanket to rest your head on
- 1 blanket to cover up
- 2 smaller cushions to support the back

☑ Preparation for the Relaxation Unit

Your participants should wear comfortable clothing and loosen them when they get into the relaxation position. Unpleasant tension or pressure points lead to readjustments in the middle of the relaxation sequence. This will only bring unnecessary unrest into the room and possibly disrupt your narrative. You should recommend that participants wear socks. Women in particular tend to get cold feet. In addition, the body temperature will drop significantly when you are in a deeper state of relaxation.

So it's advisable to offer them a blanket for comfort, even with higher temperatures.

Corpse Pose: Ideally, your participants lie on their backs in Shavasana, the Corpse Pose. It helps to relieve physical and mental tension and maintain concentration for longer sessions. This facilitates the tensing and relaxing of the entire body. To relieve the strain on your back, it may be helpful to place two smaller cushions under the knees.

Pregnancy: In advanced pregnancy, Parshva Shavasana, the Side-Lying Corpse Pose is more suitable. Your participants lie completely on the side of their body with their legs bent. Many women find a cushion between their knees to be more comfortable. The head rests on the floor, on the lower arm or slightly raised on a yoga cushion.

Back Pain: If you have back pain, the two smaller cushions should be placed under the thighs near the buttocks. This will keep your lower back completely on the floor. A folded blanket could also serve to compensate for the hollow in the lower back.

Large meditation cushions have proven themselves for severe back pain. These cushions, approximately 40 cm high, are usually used when sitting on the heels in Virasana pose. When lying down, the height is suitable for elevating the legs. Place a cushion near the buttocks, with the back of the knees at the top of the cushion. This creates an angle of 90 degrees between the upper and lower leg, which optimally supports the back. A real feeling of well-being for the tormented back.

☑ Content and Process of the Relaxation Unit

The following relaxation techniques should be included in every yoga class. Use them as follows: Methods 1 through 3 for a short initial relaxation, and Methods 1 through 5 for a longer final relaxation (deep relaxation). It's possible to adapt the individual elements to your schedule, but it's important to follow the recommended order. The section "Relaxation Techniques" explains the techniques in more detail:

1. Progressive Muscle Relaxation (PMR)

Conscious relaxation on a muscular level helps to release both physical and mental-emotional tension. This makes it easier to break away from the tensions of everyday life. This is not only the prerequisite for a more intensive body awareness, but especially for opening the gates to the subconscious. Chapter 3 presents two exercise instructions for a short and a long PMR sequence.

2. Sounds

Sing a mantra or offer a short sound bath. For a sound bath, use only a few but harmonious sound elements. Singing bowls, monochords, tanpura, gong or a sansula can be used here. They interrupt the inner dialogue and focus the mind on what is happening in the moment. They are also ideal preparation for a Guided Imagery Journey because the mind reacts very receptively to calming and harmonious sounds. Such sounds often create sound images that invite you to take an inner journey. That's why the instruments can also effectively support a Guided Imagery Journey. Only use high tones (singing bowls for the head area, cymbal bells) as a clear signal to return from the state of relaxation.

3. Body Scan and Quick Relaxation
Consciously observing the sensations of the body can also be part of the Guided Imagery Journey. If this is not included, carry out a body scan first. When doing a Body Scan or Quick Relaxation, it is important to start with the feet and end with the head. This promotes concentration because a relaxation session as part of a yoga class should not be an aid to falling asleep. In chapter 3 you will find an exercise instruction for the Body Scan and Quick Relaxation.

4. Guided Imagery
The Guided Imagery Journey can be adapted to the specific theme of your yoga class. Maybe you want to give participants stimulating impulses or improve their mood. Guided Imagery Journeys free the mind from everyday thoughts, worries, and ruminations. This invites the participant on an inner journey which includes invigorating or calming impressions, allowing them a short-term vacation, refreshing body, mind, and soul. In chapter 4 you will find a large selection of Guided Imagery Journeys.

5. Belief and Affirmation
Beliefs and affirmations can have a strong influence on our everyday world. This applies to both self-chosen messages and messages conveyed to us by others. They have an enormous influence on our values or our view of the world. If we perceive them to be true, they become part of our reality. They then influence our thoughts and actions.

Therefore, it is significant to always convey positive messages during the relaxation sequence. Avoid words like "not," "never," "none," "must," or "should." Make the sentence as short as possible and as if the desired result had already been achieved. The impact of any Guided Imagery Journey can be increased if it ends with a positive belief or affirmation. Especially when the positive message is linked to the pleasant inner images from the Guided Imagery Journey.

Visualizing messages can help anchor them deeper into the subconscious. This means they have a positive effect long after the yoga class.

Essentially, every relaxation exercise should include a sequence for returning into the moment. This can be combined effectively with a positive belief or affirmation. For this reason, you will find the "Return-to-the-moment" sequence in the instructions for the initial and final relaxation exercises in Chapter 3. Furthermore, each of the Guided Imagery Journeys presented in Chapter 4 also end with a return. Each return includes various positive affirmations.

☑ Quality of the Relaxation Unit

The quality of your relaxation unit depends on both the content and how you will deliver the content. Two factors are significant for a high-quality yoga class: first, a realistic schedule and second, the effective use of your voice.

A) Exercise Time

Your concept of the yoga class can lose its effectiveness if you are under time pressure because you have not yet developed a sense of time for the duration. When preparing the content, make sure you have a realistic schedule that you can actually stick to. Choose a balanced exercise time for your relaxation elements. This will benefit you in three ways:

- Firstly, you are not under time pressure and can easily announce the relaxation unit.

- Secondly, your participants have enough time to listen to, feel and experience your messages.

- Thirdly, at the end of the relaxation unit, there is no time left over that you would have to fill out additionally.

> For beginners, it makes sense to measure the time in advance. Set an alarm and talk through the entire relaxation sequence calmly. Allow for sufficient periods of silence for the fantasy journeys. This creates a creative space in which the imagination can unfold freely.

B) Voice and Way of Speaking

Your voice is the most important and valuable instrument in yoga classes. On the one hand, it's important to protect your voice, especially if you teach a lot of classes. Therefore, it's advisable to protect your vocal tract by speaking correctly. On the other hand, you should also pay attention to the quality of your speech, i.e., how you speak and how you phrase your sentences.

In the relaxation sequence, you cannot work with your body. Participants can only listen to your messages to be inspired and supported by them. In addition, your announcements influence both the mood in the room and in the participants' state of mind. This implies that your mood quickly affects the participants. Therefore, you should check your current state of mind at the beginning of every yoga class. A small ritual before your yoga class can help to tune in, relax or centre yourself. You will see that this not only improves the quality of your voice, but also conveys the message of calm, relaxation, or concentration more authentically.

> **Test Run:** I suggest doing a test run and making a voice recording of it. You should first write down the entire relaxation sequence and then recite it calmly. You can then listen to the voice recording at your leisure and analyze it linguistically. Check your narration for the following aspects of speaking quality, and ask at least three other people for their opinions. The perception of one's own voice is subjective and physically limited. Competent criticism and advice will help you improve the quality of your narrative in the shortest possible time.

Volume: Your voice should be neither too loud nor too quiet. In the best-case scenario, you will be able to speak reassuringly quietly but still be clearly audible. Remember that it is extremely difficult for your participants to follow very quietly spoken words. It can also cause dissatisfaction if you would like to hear and follow messages but cannot hear them sufficiently. In contrast, sounds or words that are too loud can cause stress. Tolerance to noise is greatly reduced, especially when there is strong internal tension. The higher the stress level, the more sensitive the ears react. Therefore, an appropriate and easily perceptible volume is important.

Speed: Narrate at a speed that allows your listeners to absorb your words audibly and process them internally. Words and sounds create a connection between previously experienced emotions and body reactions. Consequently, every new impulse from outside is compared with the inner world of experience. So your impulses create certain feelings, emotions and physical sensations. These are valuable experiences, but require more time under stress.

Stress also affects the body's feeling and perception of the body. If your participants are very tense or stressed internally, they need more time to absorb and classify your impulses for relaxation and to physically experience them. In addition, excessive stress or traumatic experiences can also cause excessive emotional and physical reactions. Quick instructions can lead to sensory overload, which triggers additional stress. For this reason, it is advisable to speak slowly and take appropriate pauses between sentences. Especially if you encourage sensing or feeling.

Comprehensibility: Pronounce each word clearly and avoid unclear language. Your words should be understandable both acoustically and in terms of content. Unclear expression is caused by mumbles, accents, or dialects. Likewise, phrases, idioms, or empty phrases can lead to misunderstandings. Using unclear, vague or ambiguous wording can make it very difficult to follow your instructions. Therefore, opt for shorter sentences.

Choose keywords or signal words that are understandable and comprehensible to everyone. Learn a clear and precise speaking style.

Sound: Be sure to avoid the high or even shrill voice from the head region. Prefer the more sonorous sound that comes from your chest. It is characterized by a gentler and deeper quality. Its effect is calming and relaxing. You should practice both vocal differences so that you can switch quickly if necessary. Especially when you are stressed, afraid or nervous, you may tend to have more of a head voice.

Exercise: Place a hand on your chest just below the neck. Say the mantra OM several times in a higher and lower tone. Pay attention to the different sounds and feel the vibrations in your chest. The sonorous sound causes the chest area to vibrate. Head voice puts a strain on the muscles of your vocal tract if you haven't trained it with professional singing lessons. Therefore, after speaking for a long time, you may feel exhausted, have a rough sounding or sore throat. The chest voice has a massaging effect and allows you to easily maintain the same pitch for a longer period of time. It also has an extremely calming effect on you and your listeners.

Hypnotic voice: For your Guided Imagery Journeys, work with the calming sound of a hypnotic voice. A hypnotic voice initially creates an authentic connection with the listener. A positive relationship of agreement and empathy is created. This so-called rapport forms the basis for your participants to trustingly open up, allowing them to be guided on an inner journey. They feel safe, comfortable, and understood.

The narration should be clear, distinct and in a flowing sequence. The pitch should be as stable as possible. Try to avoid emotional expression as it can cause irritation. In everyday life we use different pitches to express our mood. However, as an instructor, you should be neutral by not imposing a specific feeling. This gives your participants the opportunity to move freely in their inner world. The content of your fantasy journey offers them a framework within which they can develop. Think of a colouring template that can be designed in any imaginative way.

Chapter 2
Objective of Relaxation

All processes in nature are subject to a constant alternation of activity and rest. This means that the energy of life, embodied in the forces of nature, either expands or contracts. In the Chinese philosophy of Taoism, these dual principles are represented by yin and yang. Here, yin and yang initially form polarities, opposing yet complementary forces that are dependent on one another. They are subject to continuous change, continually emerging from one another and merging into one another. This dynamic interplay represents the driving force of life, which is reflected in the rhythms of nature. Think of the fluid transitions in the seasons, times of day and phases of the moon.

Humans, as part of nature, follow these principles, both in their circadian rhythms and in their phases of life. Over the course of the day, the inherent power grows and we develop our potential and creativity. Then it withdraws and we rest, reflect and regenerate. In the same way, a child grows up and develops its individual personality during puberty. As a young adult, you develop your potential. The mature, stable personality increasingly develops inner peace and stability. It enjoys the increased prosperity and manages its own energy more carefully. As you get older, these energies slowly withdraw inwards. It is no longer necessary to build something up. It is more about enjoying life in the here and now. In the last phase of life, you tend to rest in your centre and reflect more intensively about life experiences or leaving your body.

Activity and relaxation are equally important components of our lives. If we incorporate enough moments of rest into our busy daily routine, we will find our natural inner balance much more easily. You should also plan enough time for a nap or relaxation.

RELAXATION IN TODAY'S WORLD

Our modern, fast-paced world is mainly characterized by physical and mental activities. Brief moments of calm, relaxation and wellness treatments or relaxing holidays are becoming luxuries that we treat ourselves to occasionally. In our free time, we mainly occupy ourselves with social media, television or reading. The internet offers us information, communication and entertainment. All of this distracts the mind, but never really calms it. This leads to constant inner tension, which is inevitably transferred to the body. Illnesses that are due to chronic muscular tension are now considered widespread. Stress is one of the most common causes of work absence due to illness.

> Everyone can reflect on their attitude to life and make their own decisions to improve their quality of life.

Therefore, their inner attitude is reflected in their state of health and well-being. People who consciously choose a healthy lifestyle will actively engage with aspects such as balanced exercise, nutrition and relaxation. Your participants have already taken the first step by registering for the course. It doesn't matter whether they want to reduce stress, increase their performance or improve their health in general. The motives are not crucial, as they automatically become more aware of the needs of their body and mind through regularity. With your service, you can offer them valuable support for a balanced life.

RELAXATION TECHNIQUES

Relaxation techniques are all methods that, through regular practice, reduce physical and mental tension and improve well-being and health. The following briefly introduces the clinically proven and recognized methods, particularly to highlight their value and benefits for yoga teaching.

☑ Progressive Muscle Relaxation

The American physician Edmund Jacobson (1888-1983) developed Progressive Muscle Relaxation (PMR) in the 1930s. During his research, he recognized a connection between mental restlessness (mental tension) and physical (muscular) tension. In the classic technique, 16 muscle groups are tensed and then deeply relaxed one after the other. The resulting physical relaxation has a positive influence on the entire autonomic nervous system, including heart rate, breathing rate, and blood pressure. On a mental level, this technique leads to greater balance, inner peace, and harmony.

Yoga practice: In yoga classes, PMR is used in both the short initial and the long final relaxation phases. The conscious release of muscular tension is intended to release the mental and emotional tensions built up in everyday life. This not only interrupts internal thought loops and emotions, but also reaches the deeper layers of the psyche. Therefore, PMR is considered a precursor to deep relaxation.

☑ Autogenic Training

Autogenic training (AT) was developed from the field of hypnosis by the German psychiatrist and psychotherapist Prof. Dr. Johannes Heinrich Schultz (1884-1970) in the 1920s. It is a form of autosuggestion in which inner states of tension can be gradually released using hypnotic phrases. Autogenic Training comprises **three stages**, working first on the physical level, then on the mental level, ultimately opening the gates of the subconscious and overwriting destructive thought patterns.

Schultz's pioneering work is based on the development of self-hypnosis. Autogenic Training thus allows one to independently enter a trance-like state of deep relaxation and thereby initiate profound changes.

Basic Stage: Deep Relaxation of Body and Mind
The basic stage is designed to put the autonomic nervous system into a relaxed state. This physically calming effect also has a calming effect on the mind. With regular use, stress and tension can be reliably reduced. Therefore, the basic level alone has proven effective for sleep disorders and almost all symptoms of stress syndrome.
Yoga practice: These phrases are also commonly used in other relaxation techniques for physical and mental relaxation; they are particularly helpful in the transition into deep relaxation.

Intermediate Stage: Improving Quality of Life
In contrast to the basic stage, which focuses on the physical level, the intermediate stage aims to positively influence the mental level. The goal here is to identify deeply hidden beliefs, thought patterns, and perspectives. When positive beliefs or affirmations are repeated in a state of deep relaxation, they can override negative beliefs. Since our behaviours are often the result of our attitude and inner perspective, we can easily influence our quality of life in this way.
Yoga practice: It is important to work with inspiring messages that neither appear manipulative nor impose new thought patterns. Rather, it is important to create a framework in which participants become aware of new thought patterns. They then independently develop positive beliefs tailored to their needs and life questions. This motivation can actually bring about change.

Advanced Stage: Promoting Personal Development
While the intermediate stage focuses primarily on everyday thought and behaviour patterns, the advanced stage focuses on underlying self-perception, self-purpose and values of life.

These are the essential core questions or themes with which we consciously or unconsciously grapple. The advanced stage not only promotes personal development, but especially spiritual development.

Yoga practice: The simple, autosuggestive phrases are ideal for guided imagery and other relaxation techniques.

☑ Autosuggestion

Autosuggestion means "self-influence." This technique originates from psychotherapy and involves working with the subconscious. In a state of self-hypnosis or by repetitive self-affirmation, negative thought patterns and beliefs can be replaced with positive beliefs. However, this requires a state of deep relaxation.

Yoga practice: This technique is more effective the deeper the state of relaxation. That's the reason why autosuggestion is an essential component of initial and the deep relaxation at the end of a Hatha yoga class. Autosuggestive phrases are also found in many positive affirmations. You could incorporate them as you return from the initial relaxation phase and use them as a theme for your yoga class to deepen the effect of the asanas or breathing exercises.

☑ Guided Imagery Journeys

Working with inner images originates from psychotherapy and is called imagery techniques. This involves consciously working with the mind's imagination to process deeply hidden experiences, resolve fears, problems, or blockages, or develop inner potential. Chapter 4 explains the work with inner images in the context of Guided Imagery Journeys in more detail. Professional guided imagery, through autosuggestive phrases, becomes a powerful technique that can significantly influence well-being and quality of life.

Yoga practice: For lasting change, a state of deep relaxation is also important here. Therefore, you should follow the deep relaxation sequence suggested in this book to achieve the full potential of Guided Imagery Journeys.

☑ Deep Relaxation

Body and mind are either in a state of activity or relaxation. But our mind, or more precisely, our brain waves, determine which state we are in. The autonomic nervous system is merely the interface for the physical response to initiate the necessary hormonal and physiological processes. While the sympathetic nervous system controls the organ system during times of increased activity, the parasympathetic nervous system is responsible for the necessary rest and regeneration phases.

The states of activity and relaxation can vary in intensity and flow seamlessly into one another. The type of brain wave expresses the state, and the range within its frequency influences the intensity. The transition between brain waves creates the smooth transitions regarding our activity and relaxation. Beta waves represent our daily activity mode. Nevertheless, we can already experience a slight degree of relaxation within this frequency range if we manage to lower their vibrational frequency slightly. For example, if we focus our attention on the body or mind. The passive observer role allows us to calm our mind's activity, which directly influences the speed of beta waves. However, we only begin to reach a state of deep relaxation with alpha waves, when communication with the outside world and within ourselves comes to a standstill. You can find a comprehensive overview of how brain waves work in the section "Effects of Relaxation on Brain Waves."

Yoga practice: The effectiveness of Far Eastern healing and movement methods is based on millennia-old knowledge and experience, as well as a holistic view of the human body-mind energy structure. It is important to understand that there isn't just one movement, breathing, concentration, or meditation exercise that miraculously conjures up a deep state of relaxation. Rather, it is a deep insight in the necessity and a conscious decision. These release the necessary motivation and willpower to gradually gain control over mental activity over a long period of regular practice.

Process of Deep Relaxation

It is easy to achieve a state of deep relaxation if the following sequence is followed:

1. Release physical tension with Progressive Muscle Relaxation
2. Release mental tension with Body Scan or Quick Relaxation
3. Break thought patterns with Autogenic Training or Autosuggestion
4. Prompt new ways of thinking and behaving with Guided Imagery Journeys
5. Use positive beliefs or affirmations for inspiring impulses

☑ Yoga

The holistic effect of yoga is based on a balanced state of body, mind, and energy. These connections are explained in detail in the section "Effects on Brain Waves." In yoga, the mind is gradually guided through relaxation exercises, breathing exercises, concentration exercises, and meditation exercises. First into a relaxed state, then into a concentrated state, and finally into a meditative state. After this, the mind dissolves into the super conscious state. Yoga techniques have been clinically studied for decades and have become an indispensable part of modern healthcare.

☑ QiGong

QiGong means "working with Qi." This is achieved through specific body postures or breathing movements with deep concentration. The exercises are performed gently, slowly, and evenly. The repetition of individual poses, as well as their alternation, occurs continuously and fluidly. The uninterrupted flow promotes calm and relaxation of body and mind. The breath flows calmly, and the heart beats gently. The sequence of poses follows a rhythmic alternation of tension and relaxation, but also of movement and stillness. If these principles are observed, QiGong promotes a harmonious flow of life energy (Qi).

This corresponds to the constant change of Yin and Yang. In this way, QiGong brings the inherent Yin and Yang, and thus body and mind, into their natural balance. With regular practice, this increases physical and mental performance and resilience.

☑ TaiChi

Tai Chi (full name: Tai Chi Chuan) is an ancient Chinese movement and healing art that harmoniously connects body, mind, and soul. It is based on the principles of Qi Gong and thus of Traditional Chinese Medicine. Tai Chi regulates breathing, strengthens the heart, circulatory system, and nervous system. It also promotes well-being, relaxation, and deep concentration. The Ten Principles of Tai Chi grandmaster Yang Chengfu reveal complex connections of Far Eastern philosophy, meditation, and martial arts. Philosophical aspects such as "emptiness," "right action," "fighting spirit," and "pure consciousness" are also practiced. Deep relaxation, known as "Sung," should be mastered. It is considered a prerequisite for the inherent vitality and life energy, "Qi."

RELAXATION IN THE YOGA CLASS

In yoga philosophy, relaxation means mentally and emotionally detaching yourself from everyday activities. This calms the mind and consciously directs your attention inward. Body and mind are allowed to rest. This allows the pent-up inner tensions to be released in a very short time. Just a few minutes are enough to relieve typical stress symptoms such as agitation, nervousness, inner restlessness or tension. The relaxation sequences presented here will put your participants into a state of deep and pleasant relaxation within a few minutes.

☑ Initial Relaxation

Initial relaxation is about arriving and letting go. It is an invitation to first arrive internally in the room and in the class. That is why it is so important that your participants feel welcome and comfortable. This way they can fully engage with you and the concept of your yoga class.

As soon as your participants have taken their place, lead them into a relaxed lying position. The Corpse Pose, Shavasana, is ideal for releasing physical tension while remaining awake and focused. If you have severe back pain, it should be adapted to the symptoms using blankets and pillows. For participants in an advanced pregnancy, however, the Side-Lying Corpse Pose, Parshva Shavasana, is more suitable and healthier.

At the beginning of the yoga class, many participants can be fidgety, agitated or irritable. The open position of the back relaxation position allows you to really let go mentally. This allows them to leave the stress of everyday life behind by freeing themselves from thoughts, worries or brooding. This allows the mind to adjust to and open up to new impulses. Since inner tensions are the biggest obstacles, it is advisable to first release physical tensions using Progressive Muscle Relaxation. After that, it is much easier to relax mentally through autosuggestion.

You then have the option of conveying an inspiring impulse through a positive belief or affirmation. This will be much easier to anchor it in the consciousness when you feel relaxed and receptive.

> Choose a message that fits the theme of your yoga class. This message can also serve as a theme and be linked to further information about a healthy attitude to life or lifestyle during the class.

Process of Initial Relaxation

In Chapter 3 you will find complete instructions of the following relaxation exercises. Try to keep this order during the yoga class:

1. Assume the Corpse Pose
2. Short Progressive Muscle Relaxation
3. Short Sound Bath
4. Quick Relaxation (Alternative: Body Scan)
5. Return to the Moment

Intermediary Relaxation

During your yoga class, make sure that a strenuous exercise is always followed by a deep impulse of relaxation. The following relaxation poses are particularly suitable as a soothing balance for tired muscles:

- Corpse Pose (Shavasana),
- Prone Pose (Adhvasana)
- Child's Pose (Balasana)
- Frog Pose (Mandukasana)

These relaxation poses allow you to consciously sense the more demanding poses and really let go of the physical exertion. In this way, muscular tension can be quickly released, but also new strength can be gained. This principle also applies to mental exertion. Long-term cognitive and emotional stress leads to typical stress diseases.

Stress Symptoms:
- chronic fatigue
- chronic exhaustion
- constant nervousness, restlessness or irritability
- recurring headaches
- recurring digestive problems
- painful muscle tensions
- chronic sleep disorders

For this reason, you should remind your participants to ensure that they take regular physical and mental rest breaks in their daily lives. This applies to both professional and private life. This can prevent chronic exhaustion or illness. Resistance and performance increase, and energy reserves can be recharged.

It is the healthy balance between tension and relaxation that makes it easier to manage stress.

To do this, it is advisable to make your participants aware of the first signs of exhaustion, as it is often difficult to detach themselves from tasks and allow themselves moments of rest or relaxation. A yoga course not only offers the opportunity to better understand the needs of the body and mind, but also to perceive their limits. By knowing the warning signs, they can more easily find balance in their everyday lives.

☑ Final Relaxation

While the initial relaxation helps you to turn away from everyday life for a certain period of time, the final relaxation enables a gentle return. After the yoga class, your participants can devote themselves to their daily obligations in a much calmer, clearer, and more focused manner. Deep relaxation at the end of a yoga class is essential because the yoga class itself is an active exercise program. If your participants are not able to let go during the exercises, they may leave your class with additional tension.

Another significant aspect comes from training theory:
A deep state of relaxation promotes faster physical regeneration, which helps prevent muscle soreness and stimulates muscle growth. For personal stress management in everyday life, it is also important to train your mental resilience. Yoga offers the unique opportunity to come to terms with yourself through more mindfulness and inner peace. The final relaxation is a valuable addition, as it gradually leads to a very deep state of relaxation. It is important to follow the following sequence.

Process of Final Relaxation
In Chapter 3 you will find complete instructions of the following relaxation exercises. Chapter 4 offers a large selection of fantasy journeys. Try to keep this order during the yoga class:

1. Assume the Corpse Pose
2. Long Progressive Muscle Relaxation
3. Short Sound Bath
4. Autosuggestion (Alternative: Body Scan)
5. Guided Imagery Journey
6. Return to the Moment

EFFECTS ON BODY, MIND AND ENERGY SYSTEM

The spectrum of relaxation exercises is varied and complex. It depends on which level you want to relax or which depth of relaxation you want to achieve. During your yoga class, you can address the physical, mental or energetic level, for example to release muscular tension, calm the flow of thoughts or harmonize the flow of energy.

> For your daily yoga practice, it is extremely helpful to have a good overview of the meaning and benefits of relaxation exercises. Then you can choose the exercises to suit the concept of the class. For this reason, I would like to briefly introduce you to the most important effects.

☑ Effects on the Physical Level
- relaxes muscles
- supports muscle building
- supports muscle strength
- prevents muscle soreness
- shortens regeneration time
- releases physical tension patterns
- relieves nervous restlessness
- improves sleep quality
- reduces stress symptoms
- augments performance
- augments resilience
- prevents stress symptoms
- improves stress resistance
- activates happiness hormones
- relieves stress-related digestive problems
- promotes conscious body awareness

☑ Effects on the Mental Level
- promotes well-being with relaxing alpha waves
- calms thought streams
- prevents deep states of exhaustion
- augments inner strength and stability
- augments inner peace
- augments inner balance
- augments mental resilience
- promotes acceptance and letting go

☑ Effects on the Energetic Level
- opens energy channels
- harmonizes energy flow
- recharges energy reserves
- supports faster physical regeneration
- supports faster mental regeneration

EFFECTS ON BRAIN WAVES

Our brain is constantly busy evaluating, processing and storing impressions and information, even when we are very relaxed or asleep. This neuronal activity can be measured in the form of brain waves using electroencephalography (EEG). The neurones in the brain communicate in the form of electrical impulses, and these can be represented in waves. A wave moves up and down above the zero line. The height of these deflections is given as the amplitude and the wavelength as the frequency in Hertz (Hz). Mental states and the degree of mental activity can be divided into five brain waves. An active brain is expressed in fast brain waves, while calm thought streams are expressed in slower brain waves. Yoga and relaxation exercises have a direct influence on brain waves and thus on the entire body, since the brain, as the higher-level control centre, monitors all bodily processes. When we calm the thought streams, we activate the parasympathetic nervous system in our autonomic nervous system. This not only calms breathing, blood pressure and heartbeat, but also promotes harmonious digestion as well as the essential regeneration and healing processes.

Yoga practice: If you follow Patanjali's concept of Ashtanga Yoga in your yoga classes, controlling the mind is of central importance. In his Yoga Sūtras, Patanjali describes the effect and thus the goal of yoga as follows:

> Yogaḥ Citta Vṛtti Nirodhaḥ – Yoga is the calming of the movements of the mind. (Yoga Sūtras 1.2, Patanjali)

With his eight-limbed yoga path, he left posterity a unique method for gradually controlling the mind. Together with the knowledge of brain waves, a systemic approach can be derived as to how the brain waves can be consciously transferred from an active to a slowed state. The five brain waves and the corresponding yoga approach as well as their effects on the body, mind and energy system are briefly explained below.

☑ Gamma Waves (30–100 Hz)

These extremely fast brain waves are an expression of particularly pronounced mental activity. In everyday life, they can occur in situations of high excitement, such as anxiety or panic attacks. But they also describe a state of the strongest mental activity in which the brain is working cognitively at full speed. Think of exam situations, problem-solving or moments in which you are dealing with things with great concentration. Your mind is then very alert and clear and tends to be hyperactive.

Yoga practice: This mental state is often associated with the state of concentration or even meditation. However, this is misleading because in yoga the aim is simply to focus attention on an object without actively dealing with it, until the mind even merges with the object in the state of meditation. Concentration or meditation objects only serve as support to focus and calm the scattered streams of thoughts. It is important to understand that meditation is not an active process. Rather, it is the result of immersion, more of a trance or flow state that can be experienced in deep contemplation.

☑ Beta Waves (14–30 Hz)

This frequency range corresponds to normal mental activities in which information is processed via the stimulus-response chain. Stimuli are received via the sensory organs, passed on to the brain, where they are processed and then trigger a specific reaction. Everyday communication and interaction with the environment takes place in this frequency range, from harmonious conversations to emotional conflicts such as stress or arguments.

Yoga practice: Within Ashtanga Yoga, the first two stages, **Yamas** and **Nyamas**, initially teach a virtuous and balanced lifestyle. This means that the amplitudes and speeds of the brain waves are not often in extreme ranges. Strong emotional reactions can trigger stress reactions in our body, and this harmful influence should be minimized as much as possible. The **Asanas** represent the third stage. They teach you to adopt a posture that allows you to maintain a focused, concentrated and clear mind over a longer period of time. In the fourth stage, **Pranayama**, it is possible to influence the brain waves through breath control. By consciously concentrating on the breath and breathing movements, the brain waves slow down. This is because the brain can only concentrate on one aspect - thought or breathing. If we choose to breathe, even if only for a brief moment, the flow of disturbing thoughts is interrupted.

☑ Alpha Waves (8–14 Hz)

In this frequency range, we leave the everyday activity mode and enter a state of relaxation. The speed of these brain waves is significantly lower. The physical body with all its neural and physiological processes is completely relaxed. The brain, however, remains awake, clear and receptive, although it is in a kind of standby mode. Body and mind do not have to deal with external stimuli and sensory impressions. This benefits the following four aspects:

- Firstly, we gain access to the subconscious and the memory storage. This allows us to deal with deeply hidden experiences or information that usually only influence us unconsciously in everyday life in the form of habits of thought and behaviour. Techniques such as superficial hypnosis, neuro-linguistic programming (NLP) or depth psychology are extremely successful in this frequency range. They help to recognize and resolve blocks, fears or even traumatic experiences. Healing processes at the cellular level are also favoured in this frequency range.

- Secondly, free access to the subconscious supports the development of creativity, artistic potential and even creative intelligence. Think of a serious problem for which you need a concrete solution, or a thesis that you have to complete. In the delta state, you are more likely to work feverishly on a problem-solving strategy or meticulously fill a blank sheet of paper with words on the computer. In the alpha state, you relax and automatically let go of the problem or exam stress. Think of how often we pause for a moment to relax, as an example when we try to remember where we left our car keys. Suddenly, ideas and information flash up unexpectedly. The now more open access to the memory storage helps you to use your inner library effectively.

Furthermore, your inner working memory is not blocked by other processes. This means that your brain can concentrate fully on the current question and, thanks to its increased capacity, come up with creative ideas or develop innovative solution strategies. In this way, we even promote memory performance and cognitive abilities.

- Thirdly, learning processes and learning performance improve enormously when you are relaxed. If you acquire new knowledge before going to bed or after a nap, you will be able to absorb and process more information than when you are hectic or busy. This information is processed effectively during the alpha state of sleep and stored in your long-term memory.

- Fourthly, regarding our quality of life, it is worth consciously staying in the alpha state more often. Destructive thought or behaviour patterns can be recognized, understood and replaced with healthier ones much more easily in this state. In the beta state we react - in the alpha state we create!

Yoga practice: We always achieve mental relaxation when we close our eyes and thereby give our brain a kind of short vacation because then it hardly has to deal with the outside world. Yoga, on the other hand, aims to consciously focus the flow of thoughts. The state of **Pratyahara** refers to the gathering of thoughts because in the communicative beta state the flow of thoughts is usually very restless and scattered. Since the mind is not able to concentrate on several things at once, it also constantly jumps back and forth between thoughts. We then not only feel emotionally agitated, but also mentally exhausted very quickly. In order to achieve deep relaxation, the mind and body must first be freed of tension. This is because the body and mind are inseparably connected. As a result, mental tension leads to muscular tension, particularly in the jaw, shoulders and neck. Conversely, it also means that the mind relaxes quickly when muscular tension is released. For this reason, Ashtanga Yoga begins with **Asanas**, as they quickly release physical tension and centre the mind.

In modern times, however, we also reliably work with relaxation techniques such as Progressive Muscle Relaxation. Here, a short, strong muscular tension is automatically followed by deep relaxation. But autosuggestion exercises such as the Body Scan or Guided Imagery Journeys have also proven effective in practice because we become observers of body and mind. We free ourselves from internal and external conflicts that cause tension in us. In this process of letting go, our thoughts can finally calm down. We use the power of thought that has now been freed up to consciously decide to let go on all levels.

☑ Theta Waves (4–8 Hz)

These brain waves represent the transition from deep relaxation to sleep. In the first phase of sleep, immediately after falling asleep, alpha waves dominate, which are then replaced by theta waves. The body is now very relaxed, while the brain is active. During sleep, the brain is constantly busy processing the day's experiences in the form of dreams. An exception is the dreamless deep sleep phase, in which delta waves dominate. With increasing experience, the transition from pleasant drowsiness to automatic falling asleep can be prevented, thus achieving a state of very high concentration.

When awake, the frequency range of theta waves can be reached through concentration exercises. However, it takes a lot of practice to consciously maintain this state. Occasionally, we can be surprised by so-called 'in the flow' experiences. Especially when our brain is in 'autopilot' mode and is driving a vehicle on monotonous routes without us being aware of it. Theta waves can also happen when we sink into painting, singing or writing and completely forget the world around us.

In this trance-like theta state, we lose our sense of time and space while we do something that uplifts us internally. This is when the beauty of our soul is revealed because what is inside is free to unfold outwards. Then we wake up and are surprised at what we have created that was unimaginable. The quality of concentration depends on the different wave ranges. While concentration needs to be forced in the gamma and beta states, we achieve effortless concentration in the theta state. This also gives us access to our so-called higher intelligence.

> In Ayurvedic psychology it is called **Buddhi** and is considered the centre of intuition and wisdom. With it, we make our decisions without judgment and fear. Decisions are then neither hasty nor impulsive, but rather well-thought-out, solution-oriented and sustainable.

Yoga practice: Dharana, the state of actual concentration, is the sixth stage of Ashtanga Yoga. While in **Pratyahara** thoughts still have to be actively collected and focused, in **Dharana** we can concentrate increasingly effortlessly on an external or internal object. We become mindful observers who simply take note of all aspects without identifying with them. As we penetrate deeper into the theta state, we focus less and less on our physical and mental-emotional levels. We connect with our aura, the energetic field that surrounds and penetrates our body. Now we can perceive not only our own energy field, but also that of other people. In the subsequent state of **Dhyana**, the mind opens up to the subtle level. On the one hand, we develop a subtle perception that expands our sensory perception. We become more sensitive to phenomena such as clairvoyance, clairaudience, clairgustance or clairolfactance. On the other hand, we can also experience extrasensory phenomena such as psychokinesis, telepathy and precognition or astral travel.

☑ Delta Waves (0.1–4 Hz)

These extremely slow brain waves normally occur during deep sleep. In the so-called non-REM sleep phases, the brain no longer shows any active processes and therefore represents the phase of dreamless sleep. The previously processed information and experiences are now stored in long-term memory. Deep sleep phases help the body to recover, regenerate and heal. As a result, good quality of falling asleep and sleeping through the night is crucial for our health and resilience. When awake, we cannot consciously induce a delta state. However, experienced therapists can put us into this state through deep hypnosis or trance. The patient is then not aware of what he is saying or how he is behaving and cannot remember it after the session. Nevertheless, at this level we gain access to deeply anchored, unconscious beliefs and can track down repressed traumatic experiences. Therefore, this condition can represent a valuable enrichment for the healing process of psychological or psychosomatic illnesses.

Yoga practice: When we bring the flow of thoughts to a complete standstill in **Dhyana**, deep meditation, we can enter the eighth stage of Ashtanga Yoga, the state of **Samadhi**. There are seven stages in **Samadhi**, which represent the gradual transition from ego consciousness to cosmic consciousness. While in the first stage it is still possible to distinguish between observer, object and the process of observation, in the last stage the uninvolved observer merges completely with the meditation object – until even the meditation object dissolves. Detached from matter and the linear concepts of time and space, only the higher self vibrates in harmony with the cosmic consciousness. Such a state cannot be brought about at will, but is rather the result of a continuous process of letting go of ego consciousness and the associated world views.

Patanjali describes this state as being beyond waking, dreaming or deep sleep. Interestingly, both the dreamless non-REM deep sleep phases and the **Samadhi** state are characterized by delta waves. However, there is a big difference between deep sleep and the super conscious state.

While sleep is an inactive state of consciousness, in samadhi the attention is pure and clear. The beauty of the self cannot be experienced in sleep because the consciousness is asleep. In **Samadhi**, on the other hand, consciousness expands because it is no longer blocked by everyday sensory impressions. Despite the limited possibility of reaching this state in everyday life, it is possible for us to repeatedly come into contact with our true self on the path of Ashtanga yoga. These are wonderful moments of inner harmony and peace. They allow us to glimpse our sublime nature in the state of **Sat Chit Ananda** – the perfect state of being, consciousness and bliss.

> Here man truly becomes the link between heaven and earth. Symbolized by the tree of life, he is firmly rooted in the here and now and at the same time boundlessly connected to infinity. Resting in his true nature, he has transcended knowledge into imperishable wisdom. He no longer strives for happiness and contentment, but is like a sun that shines in pure bliss and happiness.

Chapter 3
Practical Part: Relaxation

This chapter contains detailed instructions for relaxation exercises that have proven successful in yoga practice. They were designed as read-aloud texts so you can easily integrate them into your yoga class. All the exercises are taken from my book 'Sitting Yoga – 30 Mini Workouts for Work & Leisure'. In this standard work, you'll find a variety of asanas, mudras, breathing exercises, relaxation exercises, concentration exercises, meditation exercises, as well as exercises for the seven main energy centres and traditional exercises for self-liberation. In short, this is a fundamental work that encompasses almost all areas of yoga.

The selected exercises are suitable for both initial and final relaxation. They are individual modules that you can put together as you wish. For user-friendliness, however, I have divided them into the usual sequence of initial relaxation and final relaxation. They offer you a clear structure that you can follow without hesitation. The suggested sequence for deep relaxation is particularly well suited to the subsequent Guided Imagery Journeys in Chapter 4. This will enable your participants to utilize the full potential of the Guided Imagery Journeys. They will experience deep physical, mental, and energetic harmonization, leaving them feeling truly rested, invigorated, and refreshed.

> For optimal results, 'set and setting' are equally important. This applies to both the context and the content of your narration. Therefore, I recommend that you consider the framework conditions in Chapter 1 and be sure to practice correct speaking in advance.

RELAXATION EXERCISES IN YOGA PRACTICE

A coherent lesson plan is characterized by a clear structure. You are welcome to adjust the content to suit your preferences, with varying and inspiring elements. The following lesson structure has been proven successful in practice:

1. Initial Relaxation
2. Breathing Exercises
3. Warm-up Exercises + Intermediary Relaxation
4. Body Postures + Intermediary Relaxation
5. Final Relaxation (Deep Relaxation)
6. Meditation

Such a concept allows for a fine balance between activating and relaxing impulses. Of course, it is possible to adapt this structure to your intention. Pay particular attention to the initial relaxation. It helps to mentally detach from everyday life and concentrate on the yoga class. Alternatively, you can begin your yoga class with a short meditation. It is just as relaxing as it is inspiring and can serve as a useful thematic introduction. Meditations are particularly suitable after breathing exercises as they promote deep concentration.

Some yoga traditions deliberately schedule the breathing exercises and meditation at the end of the yoga class, after the final relaxation. The participants are then particularly focused and receptive and can achieve greater depth.

> Regardless of which structure you choose, it's important to decide on a schedule and stick to it regularly.

DIRECTIONS FOR READING RELAXATION INSTRUCTIONS

- **Text:** The unformatted text is your narration text. You can simply copy and read the text as it is. You can also adapt these texts to your needs. Chapter 1 contains valuable advice for making narrations correctly and clearly.

- **"Text!":** Texts in quotation marks are autosuggestive phrases or affirmations. Such sentences should be spoken empathetically and word for word.

- *Text:* Text written in italics gives you advice for the narration, such as the duration of time to maintain muscular tension or to feel body sensations.

- **Order:** The readings for initial relaxation and final relaxation (deep relaxation) are arranged in the recommended order. This allows you to read the texts one after the other.

READ-ALOUD TEXTS FOR INITIAL RELAXATION

1. Corpse Pose

Duration of breath observation: 10 breaths

Lay completely relaxed.
Arms and legs open.
Feet fall to the side.
Armpits are getting air.
Palms face upward.
Fingers are relaxed.
Shoulders and neck are relaxed.
Tongue rests loosely in the mouth.
Jaw is relaxed.
Forehead is relaxed.
Eyes are closed.
Eyes are relaxed.
Gently turn your head from side to side.
Return to the middle position.

Breath Observation:
Observe your breath. The breath flows in and out through your nose. Observe the breathing movement of your torso. When you breathe in, it rises – when you breathe out, it falls.

Alternative:
Observe your breath. The breath flows in through your nose and out through your mouth. Observe the breathing movement of your abdomen and chest. When you breathe in, your chest and abdomen rise; when you breathe out, they fall.

2. Short Progressive Muscle Relaxation

A) Tension Building
Duration of tension: 10 seconds

Build up tension throughout the body.
Build up a slight tension.
Bring your legs and feet together.
Bring your arms toward your torso.
Pull your toes toward your knees.
Lift your pelvis and tense your buttocks, legs, and back.
Draw your abdominal wall down.
Lift your chest, make fists, and tense your upper arms.
Pull your shoulders toward your ears.
Open your mouth wide, stick out your tongue, and look up.

B) Maintaining Tension
Duration of tension: 5–10 seconds each

Increase to a moderate tension throughout your entire body.
Increase to a maximum tension throughout your entire body.

C) Relaxation
Duration of relaxation: 10–30 seconds

Consciously relax all parts of your body:
Arms and legs are open.
Feet fall to the side.
Armpits are getting air.
Palms face upward.
Fingers are relaxed.
Shoulder and neck are relaxed.
Tongue rests loosely in the mouth.
Jaw is relaxed.
Forehead is relaxed.
Eyes are closed.
Eyes are relaxed.

3. Quick Relaxation

A) Quick Relaxation of Individual Body Parts
Repeat the phrases as follows:
"I relax my toes and feet!" ***(2 times)*** –
"My toes and feet are relaxed!" ***(1 time)***

Mentally repeat the following phrases:
"I relax my toes and feet!" –
"Toes and feet are relaxed!"

"I relax my ankles and calves!" –
"Ankles and calves are relaxed!"

"I relax my knees and thighs!" –
"Knees and thighs are relaxed!"

"I relax my buttocks and pelvis!" –
"Buttocks and pelvis are relaxed!"

"I relax my belly and chest!" –
"Belly and chest are relaxed!"

"I relax my lower and upper back!" –
"Lower and upper back are relaxed!"

"I relax my neck and shoulder!" –
"Neck and shoulder are relaxed!"

"I relax my upper arms!" –
"Upper arms are relaxed!"

"I relax my elbows and forearms!" –
"Elbows and forearms are relaxed!"

"I relax my wrists and hands!" –
"Wrists and hands are relaxed!"

"I relax my jaw and tongue!" –
"Jaw and tongue are relaxed!"

"I relax my cheeks and nose!" –
"Cheeks and nose are relaxed!"

"I relax my eyes!" –
"Eyes are relaxed!"

"I relax my forehead!" –
"Forehead is relaxed!"

B) Quick Relaxation of all Body Parts
Mentally repeat the following phrases:
"I relax my whole body!" *(2 times)* –
"My whole body is relaxed!" *(1 time)*

3. Alternative: Body Scan

A) Perception of the individual body parts
Time to feel each phrase: 3–5 seconds

Mentally repeat the following phrases:
"I feel my toes and soles of my feet."
"I feel my ankles and calves."
"I feel my thighs and knees."
"I feel my pelvis and buttocks."
"I feel my stomach and lower back."
"I feel my chest and upper back."
"I feel my upper arms and forearms."
"I feel my palms and fingers."
"I feel my shoulders and neck."
"I feel my jaw and tongue."
"I feel my eyes and forehead."
"I feel my head and scalp."

B) Journey through the Body
Time to sense: 30–60 seconds

Mentally travel through your body.
Feel your entire body, from your feet up to your head.

C) Whole-body awareness
Time to sense: 30–60 seconds

Feel all parts of your body simultaneously.

4. Return to the Moment

Take two or three deep breaths.
Stretch and extend your entire body.
Slowly open your eyes and smile at yourself.

Mentally repeat the following affirmations:
"I am completely relaxed!"
"I am in the here and now!"
"I AM COMPLETELY RELAXED AND AT EASE!"

READ-ALOUD TEXTS FOR FINAL RELAXATION (DEEP RELAXATION)

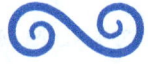

1. Corpse Pose
Duration of breath observation: 10 breaths

Lay completely relaxed.
Arms and legs open.
Feet fall to the side.
Armpits are getting air.
Palms face upward.
Fingers are relaxed.
Shoulders and neck are relaxed.
Tongue rests loosely in the mouth.
Jaw is relaxed.
Forehead is relaxed.
Eyes are closed.
Eyes are relaxed.
Gently turn your head from side to side.
Return to the middle position.

Breath Observation:
Observe your breath. The breath flows in and out through your nose. Observe the breathing movement of your torso. When you breathe in, it rises – when you breathe out, it falls.

Alternative:
Observe your breath. The breath flows in through your nose and out through your mouth. Observe the breathing movement of your abdomen and chest. When you breathe in, your chest and abdomen rise; when you breathe out, they fall.

2. Long Progressive Muscle Relaxation

A) Tension in each part of the body
Duration of tension: 3–5 seconds each

1. Lift the right leg. Draw the toes towards the knee.
   Feel light tension.
   Increase to medium tension.
   Finish with maximum tension.
   Release the tension.

2. Lift the left leg. Draw the toes towards the knee.
   Feel light tension.
   Increase to medium tension.
   Finish with maximum tension.
   Release the tension.

3. Raise your pelvis, tighten your buttocks and back.
   Feel light tension.
   Increase to medium tension.
   Finish with maximum tension.
   Release the tension.

4. Lift your chest, tighten your back.
   Feel light tension.
   Increase to medium tension.
   Finish with maximum tension.
   Release the tension.

5. Tighten your right arm and form a fist.
   Feel light tension.
   Increase to medium tension.
   Finish with maximum tension.
   Release the tension.

6. Tighten your left arm and form a fist.
   Feel light tension.
   Increase to medium tension.
   Finish with maximum tension.
   Release the tension.

7. Stretch your neck, raise your arms and spread your fingers.
   Feel light tension.
   Increase to medium tension.
   Finish with maximum tension. Release the tension.
8. Pull the facial muscles towards the nose.
   Feel light tension.
   Increase to medium tension.
   Finish with maximum tension. Release the tension.

B) Tension of the whole body
Duration of tension: 5–10 seconds each

First build up a slight tension:
Move your feet towards your knees.
Raise your pelvis and tighten your back and belly.
Lift your chest and tighten your arms.
Stretch your neck and spread your fingers.
Open your mouth and stick out your tongue.
Look up with your eyes wide open.
Increase to a moderate tension.
Increase to a maximum tension.
Hold the tension – hold – hold and release.

C) Relaxation of the whole body
Duration of relaxation: 10–30 seconds

Consciously relax all parts of the body:
Arms and legs are open.
Feet fall to the side.
Armpits are getting air.
Palms face up
Fingers are relaxed.
Shoulder and neck are relaxed.
Tongue lies loosely in the mouth.
Jaw is relaxed.
Forehead is relaxed.
Eyes are relaxed.

3. Autosuggestion "Let Go and Fly"

A) Journey through the body
Duration for feeling: 30–60 seconds

Travel mentally through your body.
Feel all parts of your body, from the feet to the head.

B) Sensation of weight
Repeat the phrases: 3–5 times

Develop a mental sensation of weight.
Repeat mentally the following phrases:
"My entire body is as heavy as a stone!"
"My body is so heavy that it sinks to the ground!"

C) Sensation of lightness
Repeat the phrases: 3–5 times

Develop a mental sensation of lightness.
Repeat mentally the following phrases:
"My entire body feels as light as a feather!"
"My body is so light, it levitates above the ground!"

D) Sensation of heaviness and lightness
Repeat the phrases: 3–5 times
Read the phrases alternately (→).

Alternately feel heaviness and lightness.
Repeat mentally the following phrases:
"My body is heavy!" → "My body is light!"
"My body is sinking lower and lower!" → "My body is levitating!"
"My body is free and I let it fly!"

Chapter 4
Practical Part:
Guided Imagery Journeys

Fantasy journeys are an imaginative technique within the field of relaxation. The use of human imagination and fantasy creates a feeling of well-being, which also relieves physical and mental tension. Our imagination enables us to create inner images, hence the term "imagination." These inner images reveal our wishes and dreams, reflect everyday events, or bring memories to life. We experience this daily in our inner dialogues, rumination, fears, and daydreams.

Imagination is closely linked to fantasy, as we can change the inner reality created at will. The fascinating and appealing thing about this is that imagination and fantasy are virtually limitless. Whether we indulge in hopeful daydreams or dreams of the future, create concrete visions, develop strategies, or create surreal fantasy worlds, inner reality opens up a space for creativity, retreat, refuge, or self-protection. Psychotherapy has long recognized the value of imagination and uses it reliably, for example, in behavioural or trauma therapy. In psychotherapy, imagination exercises can help resolve inner conflicts, manage fears or panic attacks, or process stressful experiences. It's especially important for you as a course leader to be aware of your limits.

> Yoga classes support your participants in managing stress by encouraging them to relax and recover, as well as to lead a healthy lifestyle and aid personal development. **Please note:** Only trained therapists can professionally identify and treat mental diseases and trauma.

GUIDED IMAGERY JOURNEYS WITHIN YOGA CLASSES

Guided Imagery Journeys are an integral part of deep relaxation at the end of yoga classes. They combine the power of imagination and fantasy. Typically, you can choose between the following three goals:

Physical and mental relaxation: Your Guided Imagery Journey creates pleasant inner images and promotes soothing sensory impressions. The focus is on deep, pleasant relaxation of body and mind.

Physical and mental health: Your Guided Imagery Journey offers positive messages for coping with stress and everyday life. It promotes pleasant emotional experiences, sensitizes sensory and physical awareness, and contributes significantly to a better body image.

Subtle, energetic health: Your Guided Imagery Journey offers inspiration for becoming more aware of your own energy field, releasing energetic blockages or congestion, and harmonizing the flow of energy. The more freely life energy circulates in the energy channels, the more vital, well-being, and healthier you feel.

FORMS OF GUIDED IMAGERY JOURNEYS

Guided Imagery Journeys invite you to let go, relax and dream. In principle, any imaginative story could serve this purpose. Professional Guided Imagery Journeys, however, contain keywords used in Autosuggestion or Autogenic Training. The story determines the framework in which the mind moves, but it is the keywords that guide it in a targeted manner. In principle, a fairly simple story structure is perfectly sufficient, provided it is designed to be varied for sensory or mental-emotional perception. More complex stories follow a continuous process that leads, for example, from gross to subtle perception. In this case, attention is gradually directed from the physical to the mental to the energetic level. Everything that is seen, heard, smelled, tasted, felt or emotionally sensed becomes a milestone on the inner journey.

Perceptual Building: Imagine the structure of a Guided Imagery Journey as a building. Here you want to invite someone to explore it curiously. The theme of the story sets the framework and represents the walls of the building. A clearly defined theme therefore offers a safe framework within which the mind can move. The form of the Guided Imagery Journey determines how densely the rooms inside the building are laid out and how freely the mind can move within them. Each room represents a creative space, a sub-aspect of your journey that can be experienced. These could be different places, objects, or themes. While the corridors between the rooms guide the mind from one perceptual space to another, the stairs lead to different floors. Each floor can be viewed as a level of perception–physical, mental, or subtle. Thus, one of these levels can be explored extensively, as well as switching between levels. In a simple story structure, there may only be one or two rooms, but they are complexly designed. If the story is thematically more complex, however, the building offers many rooms. A multifaceted Guided Imagery Journey can address significantly more aspects. In this case, your story absolutely needs clear guidance. Also remember to include a clear way back to the building's entrance.

Forms of Guided Imagery Journeys: The following forms of Guided Imagery Journeys don't differentiate between beginner or more advanced levels. Rather, they are about what's needed at the time. An emotionally tumultuous mind requires a tightly-knit structure to calm, clarify, and refocus. If your participants are already very relaxed, open, and receptive after the yoga class, their minds can delve deeper and develop more freely. If the content of the Guided Imagery Journey aligns with the theme of your yoga class, your yoga class can conclude perfectly with the inner journey.

☑ Closed Guided Imagery Journeys
Here, the story is based on a tightly woven structure. The mind and senses are guided from beginning to end by clear instructions. Inner images or sensory perceptions are described as precisely as possible. This makes it easier for the listener to connect with the images and actively follow the keywords.

Typical Sentence Structures:
- "Imagine..."; "You feel..."; "You taste..."; "You hear..."
- "A fresh breeze cools your forehead."
- "You listen to the song of the blackbirds."
- "You look at the pebbles in front of you. A heart-shaped one particularly catches your eye. You pick it up. Pleasantly cool and smooth, it rests in your hand."
- "The path forks. You follow the gently curving path to your right."

☑ Semi-Open Guided Imagery Journeys
These stories are also closed Guided Imagery Journeys, but offer the mind a certain amount of freedom within the tightly woven structure. This allows the mind to decide for itself what or how it wants to perceive something.

Typical Sentence Structures:
- "Look around. What do you see? What do sense? What do you taste? What do you hear?"
- "You listen to the birds singing. Which sound do you particularly like?"
- "You look at the pebbles in front of you. One particularly appeals to you. You pick it up. How does it feel?"
- "The path forks. Which one do you choose?"

☑ Open Guided Imagery Journeys
These stories allow the mind to move completely freely. You simply open the door to the listener's perceptual space, which they can fill imaginatively. The inner journey begins with a clear theme and ends with clear signals. Short prompts can serve as guides and creative support to prevent the mind from drifting off or becoming sleepy.

Typical Sentence Structures:
- "You fly safely across the endless sky. You gaze at the landscape passing beneath you."
- "You lie relaxed in your boat. You gaze up at the sky. What do you see?"
- "Light-footed, you follow the gently winding paths of the enchanted forest. You marvel at the colourful variety of blossoms. You enjoy their enchanting scent. You listen to the birdsong."

PROCESS OF GUIDED IMAGERY JOURNEYS

Preparation: Your participants should be well-prepared to immerse themselves in the Guided Imagery Journey. The framework conditions, such as the room atmosphere and room equipment, play an important role here (see the section "Framework Conditions"):

- They feel comfortable and lie down.
- The room is at a pleasant temperature, and you offer them a blanket.
- They feel undisturbed and have enough time for their inner journey.

Relaxation: When your participants feel comfortable and at ease, they can fully relax physically and mentally. Especially after a challenging yoga class, muscular tension should be released. The mind should also calm down so they can openly engage with your story:

- Progressive Muscle Relaxation can release all muscular tension in a very short time.
- Body Scan, Quick Relaxation, or other auto-suggestive exercises can also help release physical tension. They relax the mind, making it more receptive to new stimuli and more sensitive to bodily sensations.

☑ Opening

The opening section is intended to introduce the mind to the story's theme. Recall the analogy with the building. The listener enters the building and closes the front door. Now he embarks on his inner journey. He consciously shuts out external reality and explores his inner reality.

☑ Journey

The main part lasts at least 5–10 minutes. Longer journey times allow for more and deeper experiences. The form of the Guided Imagery Journey determines how the mind can explore the perceptual spaces. For closed and semi-open Guided Imagery Journeys, ensure sufficient pauses of 10–20 seconds between perceptions. For open Guided Imagery Journey, you should offer short, guiding or inspiring stimuli every 1–2 minutes. This prevents them from falling asleep, supports focus, and prevents the mind from drifting off. Another aspect concerns the quality of perception. You want to generate positive thoughts and feelings, but negative associations may arise due to the different experience horizons of your participants. In this case, your stimuli can draw the mind's attention to pleasant perceptions. It is also conceivable that certain mental or emotional qualities are perceived for the first time. In this case, the mind may need a little support to better understand and classify the new experiences.

☑ Return

The inner journey ends with a clear return to the starting point. Think again about the example of the building. If the perceptual spaces are complex and the experiences during the inner journey are very intense and rich, the mind should be safely guided back to the building entrance. This is especially true if your participants are working with their subconscious. This is a conscious return to external reality. Send clear signals for a gradual return. Allow your participants sufficient time for this. If the return is part of the story, it's advisable to use the same words as at the beginning of the journey. This makes the starting point more clearly identifiable.

So that your participants can return to their everyday lives awake, clear, and focused, they should be guided gently but firmly back to external reality. Body and mind are then receptive to everyday activities again. They should not leave your yoga room in a drowsy mood or in an intermediate state between inner and outer reality. It is important to end the deep relaxation with clear closing signals. This will enable your participants to achieve a complete return to their everyday perception. You bear a certain responsibility here, especially if the experiences were very intense.

> **Please note:** Your participants should be able to drive a vehicle without difficulty after the yoga class.

Process of Return

The following procedure for the physical and mental return to the here and now has proven to be effective in practice.

1. **Physical Activation:** First, feel your fingers and toes and move them slowly. Then stretch and extend your entire body.

2. **Mental Activation:** Smile to yourself internally and repeat the following affirmations in the given order.

    "I'm fine!"
    "I'm completely relaxed!"
    "I'm in the here and now!"

3. **Positive Message for Everyday Life:** Open your eyes and repeat a key affirmation that aligns with the theme or content of your guided imagery.

    Examples:
    "I feel light and free!"
    "I feel warm and comfortable!"
    "I feel cool and refreshed!"
    "I feel clear and liberated!"
    "I feel recharged and energized!"
    "I love life, and life loves me!"

Conclusion: Every Guided Imagery Journey can be a profound experience for your participants. In every inner journey, they encounter themselves and learn about aspects of their personality. Suddenly, entrenched feelings or emotions surface and create unrest. But this also presents the opportunity for a new perspective, toward their resolution. Destructive thought or behaviour patterns can be recognized and resolved. They may receive inspiration for coping with everyday life and stress.

For most participants, deep relaxation will be an oasis of retreat and recovery. Here, they can confidently let go of everything and withdraw into themselves. In today's hectic and demanding modern world, they experience true moments of relaxation. However, relaxation must be learned, and holistic relaxation is a new experience for many. A balanced yoga program with holistic relaxation elements offers real added value for the health, well-being and quality of life of your participants.

DIRECTIONS FOR READING GUIDED IMAGERY JOURNEYS

- **Text:** The unformatted text is your narration. Feel free to copy and read aloud. Of course, you can adapt this text to your needs. Chapter 1 contains valuable tips for creating an effective narration.

- **– :** A dash marks a short pause, giving your participants the opportunity to sense, feel, or perceive. The entire Guided Imagery Journey should generally be read very slowly.

The following texts should be emphasized and read out verbatim:

- *Text:* Texts written in italics are autosuggestive phrases based on the basic stage of Autogenic Training.

- <u>Text:</u> Underlined texts are also autosuggestive phrases, which work with the intermediate and advanced stage of Autogenic Training.

- **"Text!":** Texts in quotation marks are positive affirmations.

READ-ALOUD TEXTS OF GUIDED IMAGERY JOURNEYS

Body of Light

You are surrounded by <u>warm, soft</u> light –
there is light everywhere – beautiful, radiant light –
make the light a certain colour –
the light engulfs your body – above – below – everywhere –
it is soothing – your breathing becomes very calm –
you feel peaceful, warm, and comfortable

Warm light flows into your body –
flowing into your feet and ankles –
feet and ankles are glowing –

flowing into your calves and shins –
calves and shins are glowing –

flowing into your knees and thighs –
knees and thighs are glowing –

flowing into your pelvis and buttocks –
pelvis and buttocks are glowing –

flowing into your stomach and chest –
stomach and chest are glowing –

flowing into your lower and upper back –
lower and upper back are glowing –

flowing into your shoulder and neck –
shoulder and neck are glowing –

flowing into your arms and elbows -
arms and elbows are glowing -

flowing into your palms and fingers -
palms and fingers are glowing -

flowing into your head, skin and hair -
head, skin and hair are glowing -

<u>The light flows through your whole body -</u>
<u>warm, calming light</u> -
your body is pure light -
your body is glowing -

*A feeling of deep peace engulfs you - serenity -
you are at ease and relaxed -*

Return: Take two or three deep breaths. Stretch and extend your entire body. Slowly open your eyes and smile to yourself. Repeat in your mind the following affirmations:

"I am thoroughly relaxed!" –
"I am in the here and now!" –
"I AM FULL OF LIGHT AND LOVE!"

Journey on a Cloud

You lie on a cloud –
on a white, soft, billowing cloud –
your body is <u>weightless</u> – <u>everything is airy</u> –
your head is light – shoulders and neck – very light –
back and pelvis – arms and legs – hands and feet –
<u>as light as a feather</u> –

<u>The cloud gently touches your bare skin</u> –
it tickles and tingles pleasantly –
you stretch out and sigh – snuggle a little deeper –
<u>you feel warm and safe</u> –

The sun warms you –
covers your body –
you feel warm and cozy –

A light wind breezes in, now and then –
refreshes your eyes and forehead –
your mind is aware and clear –

<u>With a deep breath, you let go of all burdens</u> –
with each breath, you become <u>lighter and lighter</u> – <u>weightless</u> –
while inhaling, you feel your body –
while exhaling, you feel it floating, higher and higher –
inhaling, you feel – exhaling, you float –
inhaling, you feel – exhaling, you float –

You float weightless into the infinite sky –
you feel <u>boundless and free</u> –
nothing hinders you –

Completely quiet up high –
silence all around you –
silence within you –
you relish the silence –

Your breathing is calm and even –
you feel peace – silence – peace – silence –

Return: Take two or three deep breaths. Stretch and extend your entire body. Slowly open your eyes and smile to yourself. Repeat in your mind the following affirmations:

"I am thoroughly relaxed!" –
"I am in the here and now!" –
"I FEEL LIGHT AND FREE!"

Sand Bath

Imagine yourself lying in the warm, smooth sand –
feeling the fine sand against your bare skin –
it is soft and warm –
the warmth flows through your entire body –

You snuggle comfortably deeper into the sand –
feeling it pleasantly cool in your hands –
it trickles gently through your fingers –
you play lazily with the small grains –
feeling them gritty, pointed or round –

You are completely calm and heavy, delightfully heavy –
the heaviness flows through your entire body –
you feel heavy in your head –
in your shoulder and neck – in your arms and hands –
in your back and pelvis – in your legs and feet –
as you exhale, you become heavier and heavier –
everything is heavy –

The sand carries you, warms you –
envelops you – very tenderly –

you feel warm and comfortable –
your breath flows calmly and evenly –
you are entirely calm, relaxed, and at ease –

Return: Take two or three deep breaths. Stretch and extend your entire body. Slowly open your eyes and smile to yourself. Repeat in your mind the following affirmations:

"I am thoroughly relaxed!" –
"I am in the here and now!" –
"I AM COMPLETELY RELIEVED AND RELAXED!"

Summer Night

You are lying in a hammock –
enjoying the silence of a mild summer night –
only the crickets and cicadas are chirping –
a nighttime concert – just for you –
now and then an owl calls –
<u>otherwise silence – silence expands in you</u> –

<u>Your thoughts become sleepy</u> – like your body –
it lies comfortably here – wrapped in soft cotton –
<u>it envelops you protectively, like a cocoon</u> –

You let go of the hustle and bustle of the day –
your arms and legs loosen – then your shoulders and neck –
contentedly, you let go of everything – you are completely relaxed –

The sweet odour of night-scented flowers embraces you –
you inhale it deeply –

Playfully, you begin to sway –
very gently – then swing vigorously –
<u>you feel free – exuberant and free, like a child</u> –

You return to your inner peace –
look to the cloudless, dark-blue sky –
it's a starry night – the moon shines mystically –
you gaze in awe at the countless lights –
millions of sparkling stars and planets –
Do you recognize the constellations? –

An airplane flies by, blinking –
there, a satellite, and it's already passing by –
<u>like your thoughts – they appear and they pass by</u> –
<u>thoughts appear – thoughts pass by</u> –

Suddenly, you see a shooting star –
Make a wish! –

Return: Take two or three deep breaths. Stretch and extend your entire body. Slowly open your eyes and smile to yourself. Repeat in your mind the following affirmations:

"I am thoroughly relaxed!" –
"I am in the here and now!" –
"I AM HAPPY AND AT EASE!"

Chakra Journey

You feel your body – warm and comfortable –
you breathe calmly and evenly – calmly and evenly –
you feel tranquillity within you – you are completely at peace –
completely relaxed and at ease –

Energy flows into your feet – feel your feet –
as you inhale, <u>warm, golden energy</u> flows into the soles of your feet –
as you exhale, the energy radiates in all directions –

The energy flows to your pelvic floor – feel your pelvic floor –
as you inhale, <u>warm, golden energy</u> flows to your pelvic muscles –
as you exhale, the energy radiates in all directions –

The energy flows to your pelvis – feel your pelvis –
as you inhale, <u>warm, golden energy</u> flows to your sacrum –
as you exhale, the energy radiates in all directions –

The energy flows to your belly – feel your belly –
as you inhale, <u>warm, golden energy</u> flows to your navel –
as you exhale, the energy radiates in all directions –

The energy flows to your chest – feel your heartbeat –
as you inhale, <u>warm, golden energy</u> flows to your heart –
as you exhale, the energy radiates in all directions –

The energy flows to your neck – feel your neck –
as you inhale, <u>warm, golden energy</u> flows to your throat –
as you exhale, the energy radiates in all directions –

The energy flows to your forehead – feel your forehead –
as you inhale, <u>warm, golden energy</u> flows between both eyebrows –
as you exhale, the energy radiates in all directions –

The energy flows to your crown – feel your crown –
as you inhale, <u>warm, golden energy</u> flows to the top of your head –
as you exhale, the energy radiates in all directions –

As you inhale, <u>warm, golden energy</u> flows from your feet to the crown – as you exhale, <u>warm, golden energy</u> flows from the crown to the feet –

Flowing from your feet to the crown –
from the crown to the feet –
feet to crown – crown to feet
feet to crown – crown to feet

Return: Take two or three deep breaths. Stretch and extend your entire body. Slowly open your eyes and smile to yourself. Repeat in your mind the following affirmations:

"I am thoroughly relaxed!" –
"I am in the here and now!" –
"I AM CONNECTED WITH COSMIC ENERGY!"

Full Moon

Imagine a warm summer night –
you are sitting on the shore of a lake –
millions of tiny stars sparkle in the black night sky –
and frame a large, clear full moon –
you gaze at the smooth surface of the water –
the full moon is mystically reflected –
a shimmering white bridge to its power –

The moonlight covers your face, touches your heart –
your hands rest on your heart –
<u>you are close to yourself – you feel –</u>
<u>you are completely yourself</u> –

You gaze at the moon – sinking deeper and deeper –
<u>you feel the loving connection to yourself</u> –
you inhale deeply and contentedly –
you smile to yourself inwardly –
as you exhale, pure love flows to your heart –

The powerful full moon symbolizes new beginnings –
<u>you trust the magic of new beginnings</u> –
What is it you want to begin? –

In the clear water, you recognize yourself –
<u>accept yourself as you are</u> –
What is it you want to accept? –

Connect with your lunar energy centre –
feel this chakra above your right eyebrow –
there, a spring of clear, pure water emerges –
it flows gently through your entire body –
<u>it cleanses and frees you</u> –
What is it you want to release? –

Return: Take two or three deep breaths. Stretch and extend your entire body. Slowly open your eyes and smile to yourself. Repeat in your mind the following affirmations:

"I am thoroughly relaxed!" –
"I am in the here and now!" –
"I AM THE CREATOR OF MY LIFE!"

Yoga Nidra

Travel quickly through all parts of your body in your mind. While doing this, mentally repeat the name of the named body part and feel that body part as intensely as possible.

Each body part individually:
Feel your right hand, feel your thumb, index finger, middle finger, ring finger, little finger, palm, back of the hand, wrist, forearm, elbow, upper arm, shoulder joint, and armpit.

Feel your left hand, feel your thumb, index finger, middle finger, ring finger, little finger, palm, back of the hand, wrist, forearm, elbow, upper arm, shoulder joint, and armpit.

Feel your rib cage, feel your right breast, left breast, sternum, navel, belly, pelvis, front of the thighs, knees, shins, ankles, both big toes, second toes, third toes, fourth toes, fifth toes, all toes at once.

Feel all your toes, the soles of your feet, ankles, calves, backs of your knees, backs of your thighs, buttocks, lower back, mid-back, upper back, spine, shoulder blades, and shoulder.

Feel your neck, back of your head, top of your head, forehead, eyebrows, eyes, cheeks, nose, ears, upper jaw, lower jaw, tongue, teeth, and chin.

All body parts together:
Feel the right arm – the left arm – feel both arms –
feel the right leg – the left leg – feel both legs –
feel both arms – both legs –
feel both arms and legs together –

Feel the pelvis – belly – chest –
feel the entire front of the body –
feel the buttocks – back – spine – shoulder –
feel the entire back of the body –
feel the front and back of the body –
feel the front and back of the body –

Feel the head, its skin and hair – feel head, skin and hair –
feel the entire head – feel the entire head – the entire head –

Feel the head and body – feel the head and body –
head and body – head and body –
feel the entire body – feel the entire body –
the entire body – the entire body –

Return: Take two or three deep breaths. Stretch and extend your entire body. Slowly open your eyes and smile to yourself. Repeat in your mind the following affirmations:

"I am thoroughly relaxed!" –
"I am in the here and now!" –
"I RELEASE MYSELF FROM EVERYTHING!"

Sacred Temple

You find yourself in a sacred temple –
sitting in meditation pose – looking around –
you see a magnificent marble floor – majestic columns –
colourful light flows through windows – incredible wood carvings –
walls decorated with divine images – sacred symbols –

<u>Everything is silent – silence surrounds you – silence within you</u> –
you look up to your forehead – <u>soothing darkness envelops you</u> –
you look deeper and deeper into the darkness –
What is it you see? –

Your attention moves to the crown of your head –
there is light – so much light –
<u>you wear a crown of pure light</u> –

*You feel your breath – very shallow – barely aware –
it flows to the crown of your head – breath and crown are one –
with each breath, the crown of light expands –
more and more – into infinity –*

<u>You feel one with the universe</u> –
<u>sacred silence – you are the silence</u> –
you expand – into endless space –
sacred silence – endless space –
silence – space – silence – space –

You return to the temple –
you contemplate the images and symbols –
one is very captivating –
<u>you smile knowingly – full of insight</u> –

Return: Take two or three deep breaths. Stretch and extend your entire body. Slowly open your eyes and smile to yourself. Repeat in your mind the following affirmations:

"I am thoroughly relaxed!" –
"I am in the here and now!" –
"I FEEL INNER SERENITY!"

Enchanted Forest

You are standing in front of a giant portal with two golden leaves –
richly decorated with filigree ornaments and mysterious symbols –
you open the portal – and enter immediately a magical forest –

<u>The time stands still – the magic surrounds you</u> –
you gaze around in amazement –
in the mystical fog – you see marvellous branches –
sweet-smelling flowers – luminous moss –
a secret place for fairies and elves –
full of sparkling crystals – and glitter dust –

Magnificent giant trees line a glowing path –
you follow it, light-hearted and joyful –
you feel soft moss tenderly under your bare feet –
with every step, the green ground begins to glow –
followed by glittering sparks –
they whirl around your feet –
mingling with dancing fairy lights –
and colourful butterflies –
magical flowers in the undergrowth turn curiously toward you –
an overwhelming superbloom –
multiple forms in a rainbow of colours –

One flower attracts you magically –
you marvel at its stunning details –
you gently touch its velvety petals –
they vibrate ever so gently –
its exhilarating scent tickles your nose –
you inhale deeply –
<u>and suddenly, you feel light and at ease</u> –
<u>a feeling of deep peace and pure joy</u> –
<u>Everything is good!</u> –

You hear a beautiful melody – it taunts you –
you follow the winding path to a circular clearing–
in the middle of a colourful meadow of flowers – a small pond –
its water mesmerize you – you approach in awe –

*The surface is entirely still and clear – like your mind
you are smiling looking at your reflection*

A beautiful lotus flower floats before you –
it glows from within –
you are intrigued and observe a seed –
deeply hidden, small and golden –
you sink into its delicate shimmer – deeper and deeper –
you recognize yourself – you see the true beauty of yourself

Return: Take two or three deep breaths. Stretch and extend your entire body. Slowly open your eyes and smile to yourself. Repeat in your mind the following affirmations:

"I am thoroughly relaxed!" –
"I am in the here and now!" –
"I SEE THE BEAUTY OF MY SOUL!"

Bird's-eye View

You sit in a quiet park –
you gaze longingly at the sky –
you want to escape everyday life –
<u>you want to be free, like a bird – without limitations</u> –

You spread your arms wide –
they become wings – mighty, strong wings –
you flap them, and suddenly, you take off –
soaring higher and higher –
the trees and meadows beneath you become very small –
<u>you feel weightless – light and majestic</u> –

You glide over the rooftops of your city –
you look at the hustle and bustle in the streets and squares –
<u>you are a silent observer – just an observer</u> –

It is liberating to observe everything from the outside –
<u>you enjoy the view – the overview – the bird's-eye view</u> –
you change direction – you leave your everyday life behind –
you fly to a place of your dreams –

The landscape glides beneath you –
you follow a sparkling river –
it meanders lazily between fields and meadows –
it flows calmly, like your breath – calm and steady –

You feel the wind beneath your wide wings –
it carries you safely – you glide weightlessly –
<u>your thoughts are lost in the wind</u> –
<u>your mind is clear and open</u> –

You observe the landscape's beauty –
from a magnificent perspective –
<u>everything is tiny and unimportant</u> –

Above you, the endless sky –
a bright blue, boundless sky –

<u>You feel free – freedom above you –</u>
<u>freedom below you – freedom within you</u> –

Return: Take two or three deep breaths. Stretch and extend your entire body. Slowly open your eyes and smile to yourself. Repeat in your mind the following affirmations:

"I am thoroughly relaxed!" –
"I am in the here and now!" –
"I SUSTAIN AN OVERVIEW AND A BROAD VISION!"

Glowing Heart

You wander through an ample garden –
between wide lawns – colourful flower meadows –
across idyllic brooks, with arched bridges –
under shady trees from all over the world –
to a beautiful castle –
a castle garden with numerous arbours –
you can stroll like in the old days –
to colourful, exotic plants –
and fragrant rose bushes –
you are attracted by a magnificent rose –

A small lake invites you to linger –
you feel like sitting on one of the white benches –
you look around – colourful ducks on the grassy shore –
a swan majestically passes a fountain –
people mingling on green hills – enjoying picnics and games –
children playing – you hear their laughter –
<u>it makes you smile – everything is peaceful</u> –

You feel your heart – it laughs with joy –
<u>it expands – opens</u> –
happy memories of long-forgotten childhood days –
precious moments of your life –

You are in total harmony – <u>self-love engulfs you</u> –
you know everything is love – <u>you love, and you are loved</u> –
you feel the love – <u>unconditional, all-encompassing love</u> –
<u>your heart expands – further and further</u> –
you want to share your love with everyone –

You breathe to your heart – bright light radiates from your chest –
with every inhalation, light and love flow to your heart –
with every exhalation, you share light and love –
you send them to a loved one –
you send them to your family –
your friends – to everyone –

Return: Take two or three deep breaths. Stretch and extend your entire body. Slowly open your eyes and smile to yourself. Repeat in your mind the following affirmations:

"I am thoroughly relaxed!" –
"I am in the here and now!" –
"I SHINE IN THE LIGHT OF LOVE!"

Canoe Trip

Imagine you are sitting in a canoe -
floating leisurely on a calm river -
it meanders through a beautiful, white pebble bed -
your canoe rocks gently - quite pleasantly -
<u>you trust in the water to carry you</u> -

It is quiet here - as quiet as it is inside you -
you feel the sun warm on your bare skin -
a pleasant breeze cools your forehead -

Your hand glides through the water -
silky, it flows around your fingers - rippling the surface -
you follow them until you lose sight of them -
you listen to the water - a gentle ripple here and there -
<u>you have to listen very carefully to even notice it</u> -

The river flows slowly -
it follows its course, <u>carefree and unconcerned</u> -
you decide to do the same -
<u>simply let go of all thoughts</u> -

Glittering drops of water bubble upwards –
dissolve into a ripple –

It feels like a game –
<u>every thought becomes a drop of water</u> –
it bounces – then dissolves into a ripple –
it's an endless game –
jumping thought – dissolving ripple –
jumping thought – dissolving ripple –
the thoughts dissolve easily –
thought – wave – thought – wave –

Your mind becomes entirely tired of drab thoughts –
you lean back – look up at the sky –
you see clouds lazily passing –

<u>The gentle rocking of the canoe lulls you to sleep –
your mind becomes ever so sleepy –</u>

The water flows pleasantly slow –
barely sensible – it carries you gently and safely –

*Little by little, all tension leaves your body –
leaves your arms and legs – shoulder and neck –
back and stomach – buttocks and pelvis – eyes and forehead –
you are completely relaxed and at ease –*

Return: Take two or three deep breaths. Stretch and extend your entire body. Slowly open your eyes and smile to yourself. Repeat in your mind the following affirmations:

"I am thoroughly relaxed!" –
"I am in the here and now!" –
"I TRUST IN THE FLOW OF LIFE!"

South Sea Beach

You're enjoying a beautiful beach in the South Pacific –
the sand is warm, soft and wonderful –
you feel the warmth flowing through your entire body –
you stretch out with pleasure – nothing bothers you –

A refreshing breeze gently caresses your body –
your feet play in the deeper sand – *you enjoy the cool grains –*

Palm fronds provide shade – they sway gently in the wind –
you listen to their rustling sound – it is wondrously calming –

It's a deserted beach – the sea is calm –
small waves reach the shore with power and courage –
only to return softly to the endless sea –
an eternal rhythm – <u>of farewell and new beginnings</u> –

Your breath adapts to this timeless playing of the waves –
as the waves flow toward the shore, you inhale powerfully –
as the waves retreat, you exhale softly –
inhalation is a new beginning – exhalation is farewell

Your mind becomes still and clear – full of awe and trust –
<u>life is all about change – you need change</u> –
What do you want to end? – What do you want to begin? –

Connect your breath with your decision –
as you inhale, invite something new into your life –
as you exhale, release something old from your life –

You smile consciously at yourself – you feel hopeful and confident –
You know everything is good! –

Return: Take two or three deep breaths. Stretch and extend your entire body. Slowly open your eyes and smile to yourself. Repeat in your mind the following affirmations:

"I am thoroughly relaxed!" –
"I am in the here and now!" –
"I AM GROWING WITH THE CHANGE IN MY LIFE!"

Forest Walk

You are walking through a sunny forest –
on a warm summer day –
the sun glistens through the canopy –
it warms your face, tickles your nose –

Leaves dance in a light breeze –
it refreshes body and mind –
you take a deep breath –
you smell the earthy scent of the forest –

You walk along winding paths –
lightly on moss-covered ground –
a squirrel hops from branch to branch –
it follows you curiously –

The forest is alive –
a symphony of sounds, just for you –
you pause, listen – leaves are gentle rustling –
birds are joyfully singing –
branches are creaking in the trees –
crunching on the ground –
a mouse scurries through the leaves –
you watch it with a smile –

You continue walking –
deeper and deeper into the forest –
the trees are now closer together –
light and shadow alternate –
a sea of green surrounds you –
majestic, ancient trees line your path –

One stunning tree mesmerizes you –
you look at it in awe – a maze of branching roots –
a massive trunk – with a lush canopy of leaves –
you touch the thick, ridges of the bark –
it feels scaly and rough beneath your fingers –
you want to hug it – connect with it –

<u>You become a strong tree</u> –
your powerful roots grow deeply into the ground –
they anchor you – ground you –
your centre is strong and stable –
you stand upright, unshakeable –
above you unfolds a mighty, expansive crown –
among the light –

Your breath flows calmly and evenly –
with each breath, energy circulates through your body –
as you inhale, you feel the cool earth energy from below –
as you exhale, you feel the warm solar energy from above –
<u>you are amazed at feeling full of energy</u> –

Return: Take two or three deep breaths. Stretch and extend your entire body. Slowly open your eyes and smile to yourself. Repeat in your mind the following affirmations:

"I am thoroughly relaxed!" –
"I am in the here and now!" –
"I AM DEEPLY ROOTED IN MY LIFE!"

Summer Meadow

You are lying in lush grass – in a colourful summer meadow –
your back nestles comfortably against the cozy blanket –
your shoulders are relaxed, as are your back and pelvis –
you are lying completely still, relaxed, and at ease –

A light breeze gently sways the grass –
a cooling sensation hits your forehead –
crickets are chirping – birds singing –
a dragonfly appears, buzzing softly –
you look around lazily –
you admire colourful flowers around you –
blue, yellow, purple, white –
one special flower catches your eye –
you gaze in amazement at this wondrous work of nature –

A courageous beetle is crawling up a tall stem –
finally, it reaches the flower –
it dives joyfully into the yellow pollen –
you have to laugh because the pollen sticks everywhere –
on its short legs – its shimmering wings – its long antennae –

You look up at the sky –
you are watching airy clouds drifting by –
they are constantly changing their shape –
it makes you quite sleepy
clouds form – clouds dissolve –
clouds form – clouds dissolve –

<u>Your thoughts also form and dissolve</u> –
a thought forms – the next moment it dissolves –
thoughts forms – thoughts dissolve –
thoughts forms – thoughts dissolve –

<u>You observe the silence between thoughts</u> –
a thought forms – it dissolves – then silence –
a new thought forms – dissolves – silence
thought – silence – thought – silence –

You enjoy soothing silence – ever expanding –
<u>Everything is silence!</u> –
<u>The silence is within you – calming, comfortable silence</u> –

Return: Take two or three deep breaths. Stretch and extend your entire body. Slowly open your eyes and smile to yourself. Repeat in your mind the following affirmations:

"I am thoroughly relaxed!" –
"I am in the here and now!" –
"MY MIND IS STILL AND CLEAR!"

Waterfall

You are at the base of a waterfall. Surrounded by meter-high stones, water rolls over high boulders forming stairs. Step by step, your gaze follows the streaming water. Higher and higher, until it disappears into the imposing mountains. Where is this water coming from? You look for its source – in vain.

A tiny a trickle of water starts its journey, deeply hidden among the rocks. Flowing over millions of pebbles, making its way infallibly between towering and massive obstacles. Nothing can stop the water! It becomes a mighty, unimaginable force of nature! You feel this primal force within you, too. Nothing can stop your primal force. You feel it in every part of your body.

You reach for one of your life's dreams. It is still very small, almost tiny. But you want it to grow. It wants to mature, to gain strength. Like water, it makes its way through the inner landscape of your mind. It flows masterfully around all doubts. It searches courageously for a path between false beliefs and concepts. It conquers mighty, roaring fears and worries. Until it allows itself to fall from the steep cliff into complete primal trust.

Leaving everything old behind, your life's dream falls confidently into a prolific pool. Now, the water can rest, completely still and clear. It is at peace within itself. After its long journey, it has finally arrived. You feel this peace within yourself. You, too, have arrived – completely at peace with yourself!

You smile at all the obstacles left behind. Becoming aware that you are a never-ending source of strength, hope, and confidence. Nothing can stop you! Every obstacle will be overcome. Every stone is a milestone on the journey of your soul. Your dreams find their way, like a stream of water. Sometimes strong and unyielding, then again smart and agile. It is not the stones that shape the path – it is the power of the water. You feel your inner strength – your life force! You feel it with every heartbeat.

Return: Take two or three deep breaths. Stretch and extend your entire body. Slowly open your eyes and smile to yourself. Repeat in your mind the following affirmations:

"I am thoroughly relaxed!" –
"I am in the here and now!" –
"I AM CONNECTED TO THE POWER OF LIFE!"

Winter Landscape

You drive into a snowy winter mountain landscape on ever winding switchbacks. You leave the city and its hustle and bustle behind in the valley. You look forward to the solitude and silence of nature. It is a grey winter day. The clouds hang heavy in the sky. But soon the clouds clear. With every switchback, the sky clears, the sun bursts enticingly through. Finally, you reach the summit. You put on your snowshoes in anticipation and step on to hidden paths between the trees.

Silence surrounds you. You are completely alone. Only snow-covered trees in a white, untouched winter landscape. Above you, the bright blue sky. Everything is white, nearly blinding. You sit down in the snow for a moment, look around, and connect with the forest. You breathe in this magnificent work of art. The white surrounds you. You feel safe, like in a protective white cocoon. The forest is silent. A motionless stillness, like a still life. You feel this ease within you.

The path cuts deep into the snow. It leads you higher into gently winding curves. You step over roots, slip between trees, climb short, steep passages. You enjoy a short break. You breathe in the clear mountain air deeply – you can even taste it. You look around contentedly. You see your own tracks, and some footprints of rabbits and birds. You listen, but you hear only the sound of various trees creaking in the gentle wind and your steady breathing – otherwise, only silence. Silence around you. Silence within you. The silence invigorates you.

You continue walking slowly and deliberately. The snow crunches underneath your footsteps. All of a sudden, the trees thin out to reveal a breathtaking view point. You take in the marvellous vast, white, pristine mountains. You feel a deep inner connection with this innocent nature. The sun reflects in the snowy white. It is pure and clear – like your mind! Childlike joy breaks free. You have to laugh, loudly and releasing!

You stretch your arms out, wanting to embrace the world. You shout into the mountains, laughing at your own echo. Do it again! And again!

Laughing, you let yourself fall backward into the soft snow. You remember your childhood. Making snow angels in winter. Giggling, you move your arms and legs. You feel like a child again, free and carefree! Pleasantly tired, you pause and reflect. What do you feel? You are entirely into yourself. You feel safe in the soft snow. The wind gently caresses your face. Snowflakes gently touch your face. You stick out your tongue, catching them with delight. They melt on your tongue, it feels first cool, then warm. You could lie here forever, just being you. But it is time to head back. Slowly, you stand up, giggling as you brush the snow off your jacket and pants. You return joyfully.

Return: Take two or three deep breaths. Stretch and extend your entire body. Slowly open your eyes and smile to yourself. Repeat in your mind the following affirmations:

"I am thoroughly relaxed!" –
"I am in the here and now!" –
"I FEEL LIBERATED AND CAREFREE!"

Dear reader,

originally, this book was meant to expand on my standard yoga compendium "Sitting Yoga – 30 Mini Workouts for Work & Leisure" with a focus on relaxation. Relaxation is the foundation of every profound yoga experience! Therefore, it is important to me to emphasize the magnitude of relaxation techniques and the powerful potential of guided imagery.

I hope this book will be a valuable and inspiring addition to your yoga or relaxation classes. If you enjoy the book, I would be delighted if you would leave a short review on Amazon or a book platform of your choice to help other readers become aware of this book. You are also welcome to contact me personally. Any feedback, whether praise, criticism, questions, or suggestions, is a valuable asset to me as an author.

contact via email: alidakossack@yahoo.com
contact form on my website: www.pranacentre.ca
I look forward to hearing from you!

I thank you, dear Regina Picco, from the bottom of my heart for your patience, precision, and dedication, including the repeated revisions of the German manuscript. Our valuable collaboration and friendship have made this book project something very special. Thanks for believing in it and supporting it passionately. Translating this book, particularly the Guided Imagery Journeys, into English was a huge challenge. Thanks for your patience over the weeks, for finding with me the best possible synonyms, and for rounding off all the sentences to keep the magic of the journeys.

I would like to express my deepest gratitude to my beloved husband Sylvain Vallee for his commitment to translating my wording into English as authentically as possible.

The final English editing was entrusted to the professional hands of Peter Michael Wiebe. It is a tremendous relief for me to know that the book project has been critically reviewed.

Warm regards,
Alida Kossack

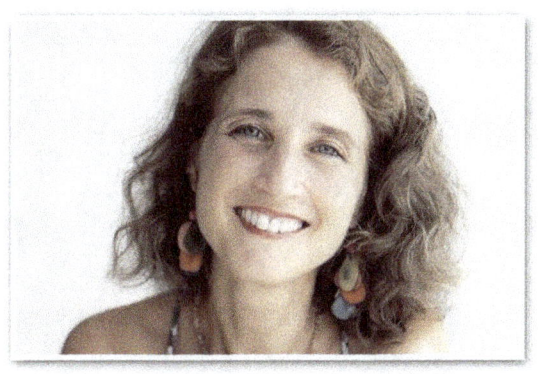

Alida Kossack, Author
Biologist (MSc), Medium

Practitioner for Progressive Muscle
Relaxation and Autogenic Training,
Yoga Therapist, Shiatsu Practitioner,
Teacher of Yoga, QiGong and TaiChi,
NLP Practitioner, Personal Fitness Trainer,
Psychological Ayurveda Consultant,
Ayurvedic Health Consultant

BOOKS BY
ALIDA KOSSACK

SPIRITUELLE FANTASIEREISEN FÜR DIE YOGASTUNDE

GEKONNT ENTSPANNEN: DER SCHLÜSSEL ZUR ERFOLGREICHEN YOGAPRAXIS
ENTSPANNUNGSTECHNIKEN ZUM BEGINN UND ENDE EINER YOGASTUNDE

informativ
Alles Wesentliche über Entspannungsverfahren,
ihre Ziele und Wirkungen auf einen Blick.
– praxisnah und benutzerfreundlich –

fachgerecht
Progressive Muskelrelaxation, Autosuggestion
und Autogenes Trainings korrekt anwenden.
– zugeschnitten auf den Yogaunterricht –

praxisnah
Detaillierte Übungsanleitungen für die Anfangs- und
Endentspannung sowie 17 inspirierende und kraftvolle
Fantasiereisen für die abwechslungsreiche Tiefenentspannung.
– einfach übernehmen und vorlesen –

Als Taschenbuch und E-Book erhältlich!

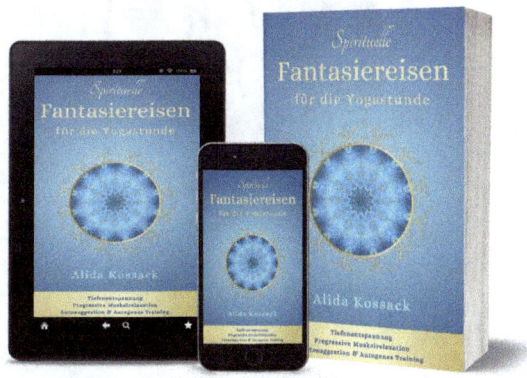

SITTING YOGA
30 MINI WORKOUTS FOR WORK & LEISURE

SITTING YOGA – ANYWHERE, ANYTIME!
NEW ULTIMATE YOGA COMPENDIUM – PRACTICAL BOOK AND LIFE GUIDE

For Beginners and Advanced Users:
Learn powerful and effective techniques for a better quality of life in everyday life. Create your own yoga program. Mini workouts for all life situations and life questions, for quick use at work or at home.

For Yoga Teachers:
A comprehensive reference book for more variety in everyday teaching, with 38 asanas, 15 mudras, 12 breathing exercises, 8 relaxation exercises, 10 concentration exercises, 10 meditation exercises, 7 self-liberation exercises, 14 exercises for the main energy centres.

Available as softcover and hardcover!

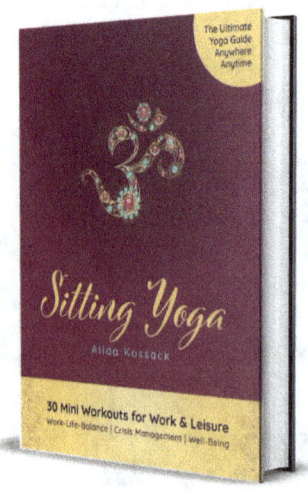

YOGA IM SITZEN
30 BLITZPROGRAMME FÜR BERUF & FREIZEIT

YOGA IM SITZEN – JETZT, HIER UND ÜBERALL!
INNOVATIVES YOGA-STANDARDWERK – PRAXISBUCH UND LEBENSRATGEBER

Für Einsteiger und Fortgeschrittene:
Erlerne macht- und wirkungsvolle Techniken für mehr Lebensqualität im Alltag. Erstelle dir dein eigenes Yoga-Programm. Blitzprogramme für alle Lebenslagen und Lebensfragen zum schnellen Einsatz am Arbeitsplatz oder Zuhause.

Für Yogalehrer:
Ein umfassendes Nachschlagewerk für mehr Abwechslung im Unterrichtsalltag, mit 38 Asanas, 15 Mudras, 12 Atemübungen, 8 Entspannungsübungen, 10 Konzentrationsübungen, 10 Meditationsübungen, 7 Übungen zur Selbstbefreiung, 14 Übungen für die Hauptenergiezentren.

Als Taschenbuch und Gebundene Ausgabe erhältlich!

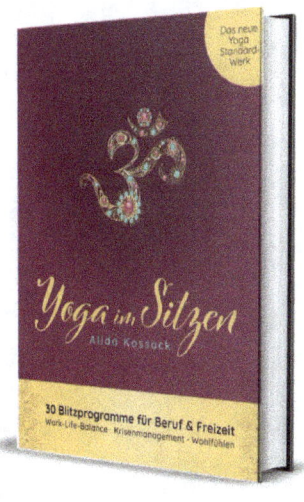

www.ingramcontent.com/pod-product-compliance
Lightning Source LLC
Chambersburg PA
CBHW050342010526
44119CB00049B/666